ADJUVENT THERAPY

ADJUVENT THERAPY

Adjuvent Therapy

Edited by

Kathy Miller
Indiana Cancer Pavillion, Indianapolis, IN, USA

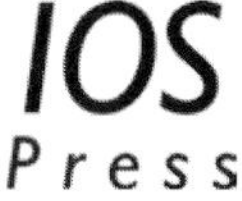

IOS *Press*

Amsterdam • Berlin • Oxford • Tokyo • Washington, DC

ISBN 1 58603 500 2
Library of Congress Control Number: 2004118303

This is the book edition of the journal Breast Disease, volume 21 (2004), ISSN 0888-6008

Publisher
IOS Press
Nieuwe Hemweg 6B
1013 BG Amsterdam
The Netherlands
fax: +31 20 687 0019
e-mail: order@iospress.nl

Distributor in the UK and Ireland
IOS Press/Lavis Marketing
73 Lime Walk
Headington
Oxford OX3 7AD
England
fax: +44 1865 750079

Distributor in the USA and Canada
IOS Press, Inc.
4502 Rachael Manor Drive
Fairfax, VA 22032
USA
fax: +1 703 323 3668
e-mail: iosbooks@iospress.com

LEGAL NOTICE
The publisher is not responsible for the use which might be made of the following information.

PRINTED IN THE NETHERLANDS

Contents

Author Index

Breast Disease 21 (2004) 1
IOS Press

Introduction

Kathy Miller
Indiana Cancer Pavillion, IN, USA

The efficacy of adjuvant chemotherapy was first demonstrated by the National Surgical Adjuvant Breast and Bowel Project (NSABP) and by the Milan Istituto Nazionale per lo Studio e la Cura dei Tumori, in the early 1970's. Prolonged follow-up of these trials confirms the lasting improvement in overall survival with the administration of adjuvant chemotherapy. In the past three decades, literally hundreds of randomized controlled trials have been performed examining the role of adjuvant chemotherapy. This mountain of often-conflicting data is best understood by examining the work of the Early Breast Cancer Trialists' Collaborative Group (EBCTCG). This meta-analysis offers the practicing physician a good sense of the broad trends in adjuvant therapy (both chemotherapy and hormonal therapy) but falls short during periods of rapid changes in available agents or approaches. We begin with two views of the Overview. Drs. Hudis and Dang highlight therapeutic advances that have not yet been incorporated into the Overview. Dr. Perez places the Overview on context, contrasting the consensus recommendations with actual delivery of therapy in the community.

While the Overview provides meaningful guidelines for the patient with an 'average risk' early breast cancer, oncologists routinely struggle with patients at either end of the risk spectrum. Dr. Green and colleagues review the use of neoadjuvant chemotherapy. Initially reserved for patients with locally advanced or inflammatory disease, they emphasize the potential advantages of neoadjuvant therapy. Equally vexing is the patient with a small primary tumor. When does the risk of toxicity outweigh the benefit of adjuvant chemotherapy? Dr. Soule takes us through the data and decisions for the patient at low risk of recurrence.

Adjuvant treatment decisions are based largely on the results of randomized clinical trials. But trials, by their nature, attempt to simplify through the rigorous application of study entry criteria. Consequently, virtually every trial is necessarily unrepresentative of the general population of breast cancer patients. In real life patients differ considerably in co-morbid conditions, psychosocial circumstances, as well as emotional and spiritual needs. In real life clinical therapy frequently requires a series of negotiations between patient and physician; the patient's needs and opinions definitely matter. The explosion of the internet makes it easier for patients to gain direct access to information and (sometimes) misinformation. Dr. Helft delves into the evolving role of the internet in patient treatment decisions.

Seasoned oncologists recognize the completion of adjuvant therapy begins a new phase in their relationship with the patient. What constitutes a 'rational' plan for follow-up after treatment? Opinions vary widely. Dr. Mollick and Carlson take us through the evidence, pointing out potential sources of bias and gaps in our knowledge. Finally, any follow-up plan must take into account the long-term complications of adjuvant chemotherapy. Dr. Partridge and Winer review the harm we may cause in our quest to improve survival.

Breast Disease 21 (2004) 3–13
IOS Press

Adjuvant Therapy For Breast Cancer: Practical Lessons From The Early Breast Cancer Trialists' Collaborative Group

Clifford A. Hudis* and Chau T. Dang

INTRODUCTION

Increased early detection and improved treatment have made clinical cure possible for more patients with breast cancer than ever before. The medical oncologist contributes to this outcome through participation in the multidisciplinary care of patients with early stage disease and by providing systemic adjuvant therapy designed to treat undetectable metastatic foci of disease. One's approach can be colored by place of training, ongoing research interests, and other biases based on data, anecdote, culture, philosophy, or even local economy. Hence, the approach to systemic treatment for patients with resectable breast cancer can vary widely. However, post-operative systemic therapy ("adjuvant treatment") is clearly effective and no doubt contributes to the falling mortality seen in many parts of the world over the past decade. This chapter reviews the meta-analyses performed every fifth year at Oxford University to provide a foundation for clinical practice, clinical trials, and for other chapters in this textbook.

OVERALL APPROACH

In most communities, potentially resectable breast cancer is treated surgically although pre-operative (neo-adjuvant) treatment is increasingly popular in some set-tings. Even without neo-adjuvant treatment (discussed elsewhere in this book), most patients with screen–detected breast cancers can be treated with breast conservation followed by radiation therapy and systemic therapy. In both the pre-operative and post-operative setting, the long term goal (cure) is the same and so the treatment selection should be similar. The complication when using pre-operative therapy is the ability to use the in-breast response to potentially tailor therapy. To date, such tailoring has not actually been proven to be beneficial but it might be in the future. Thus, the selection of systemic treatment options for individual patients should be based on the identification of the treatment most likely to result in improved survival, reduced risk of relapse, and minimal or at least acceptable toxicities. All else being equal, whether the systemic treatment is applied pre- or post-operatively is probably of limited importance except in regard to local control and surgery.

In any case, the integration of systemic therapy and local treatment – including both surgery and radiation therapy – must be considered in formulating a treatment plan. Decisions regarding adjuvant therapy should be driven by assessments of risk which are evolving as surgical techniques and biological assessments improve. For example, it is increasingly common for patients with small tumors to undergo a sentinel lymph node biopsy in lieu of the previously standard axillary dissection. Because it is critical not to miss potentially involved lymph nodes, enhanced pathologic testing is "standard" in many settings but this has added yet another uncertainty to routine clinical practice. Going

*Corresponding author: Clifford A. Hudis, M.D., Box # 206, MSKCC, 1275 York Avenue, NY, NY 10021, USA. Tel.: +1 212 639 6483; Fax: +1 212 717 3764; E-mail: hudisc@mskcc.org.

forward, oncologists will have to incorporate the additional data we are offered from this procedure into their decision making. Based upon the pathologic assessment of the tumor after surgery, the conventional and enhanced lymph node status, the patient's age and overall medical condition, oncologists can then consider more finely the various therapeutic options.

A key aspect of adjuvant therapy, as identified by the Early Breast Cancer Trialists' Collaborative Group's (EBCTCG) meta-analyses, is the property of proportional risk reduction [1–6]. The consequence of this observed therapeutic impact is that we consider the benefits of systemic adjuvant therapy to be constant in relative terms but variable in direct proportion to the size of the underlying risk. Higher risk patients will therefore benefit more than lower risk ones. At extremes of low risk, the benefits of some therapies will therefore be too modest to justify treatment but accurate risk assessment remains difficult making dogmatic approaches to therapy difficult to support. At present it is assessed by reviewing the American Joint Committee on Cancer stage including precise tumor measurement, nodal status, and prognostic and predictive factors [7], but there is every reason to believe that refinements in risk assessment using newer molecular tools including expression arrays [8] will allow for better fine-tuning in the near future. For now, however, we rely on conventional risk assessment tools. Another motivating factor in support of broad use of adjuvant therapy is the observed decline in deaths over the past decade from this disease. This suggests that while we may be overtreating some subsets of patients, overall we are providing improved outcomes through the broad use of systemic treatments [9].

THE WORLDWIDE OVERVIEW

The earliest systemic adjuvant therapy trials had limitations that made interpretation challenging. They were, in general, underpowered because of small size and modestly effective treatment interventions. As a result, they were unable to consistently demonstrate benefits or to prove their significance. Because effective systemic therapy is of broad potential impact, the EBCTCG was convened in the attempt to identify the true worth of broadly tested systemic adjuvant therapies [1–6].

Almost all effective systemic adjuvant treatments are derived from regimens with proven efficacy in the management of metastatic breast cancer. As a consequence there are only two broad categories of systemic adjuvant therapy included in the most recently published reports by the EBCTCG [1–6]. These are hormonal manipulations including ovarian ablation and selective estrogen receptor modulators (SERM's) as well as a few other less-used hormone treatments, and chemotherapy including a broad range of agents and regimens.

Adjuvant Hormone Therapy

The very first report of an effective systemic therapy for cancer was that of Beatson published in 1896 demonstrating a change in the natural history of advanced breast cancer in response to oophorectomy [10]. More than a century later the benefits of adjuvant ovarian ablation remain uncertain. The effects of adjuvant ovarian ablation on recurrence and death in women with breast cancer have been analyzed in several randomized trials. The EBCTCG has presented a recent overview with 15 years of follow-up on all trials that began before 1990 which compared ovarian ablation versus no such adjuvant treatment [6]. Data were obtained on 12 of 13 studies that assessed ovarian ablation by surgery or irradiation, all of which began before 1980. Data on the four studies that involved ovarian suppression by drugs, all of which began after 1985, were not reported in this overview. The main analyses were limited to 2102 women who were under 50 years of age. In this group of women ovarian ablation improved the recurrence-free survival by 25% in the absence of chemotherapy but only 10% in its presence, for an overall benefit by 18.5%. Similarly, the proportional improvement in survival was 24% in the absence but only 8% in the presence of chemotherapy, for an overall benefit by 18.4%. The benefit was significant regardless of nodal status. Among the 1354 women aged 50 years or older, most of whom would have been perimenopausal or postmenopausal, there was a nonsignificant improvement in recurrence-free and overall survival.

The effectiveness of ovarian ablation alone is not an open question presently. Instead questions about its worth instead of chemotherapy or especially in addition to chemotherapy remain to be answered. The former question has been addressed in several studies demonstrating equivalence between ovarian ablation, generally combined with tamoxifen, and combination chemotherapy using cyclophosphamide, methotrexate, and 5-fluorouracil (CMF) [11–13]. However, how it would compare to regimens believed to be superior to CMF is unknown and more importantly how it adds to our most effective systemic chemotherapy regimens is also unknown. In the quest to maximize the number of patients cured ,this latter question is most important. In the quest to minimize treatment-related toxicity, the comparison between chemotherapy and ovarian ablation (alone or in combination with other hormonal agents) is more important.

Tamoxifen in the Overview

The EBCTCG has published a third systemic overview on adjuvant tamoxifen treatment in early breast cancer in 1998 [5]. All randomized trials that began before 1990 involving the use of tamoxifen for any duration of treatment versus no tamoxifen were analyzed. Information was obtained on 37,000 women in 55 such trials. Nearly 8000 of these women had low or zero level of estrogen receptor (ER) measured on the primary tumor. Among the patients with ER $(-)$ tumors, the overall effects of tamoxifen were small so subsequent analyses of recurrence and mortality were restricted to the remaining 18,000 patients with ER $(+)$ tumors and 12,000 patients with ER-unknown tumors, of which an estimated 8000 would have been ER $(+)$. The proportional recurrence reductions for adjuvant tamoxifen use for 1 year, 2 years, and 5 years during 10 years of follow-up were 21%, 29%, and 47%, respectively, with a highly statistically significant trend towards greater benefit with the longer duration of treatment of 5 years $(2p < 0.00001)$. The corresponding mortality reductions were 12%, 17%, and 26%, respectively, again with a statistically significant benefit in favor of 5 years of tamoxifen treatment $(2p = 0.003)$. The absolute improvement in recurrence was greatest during the first 5 years, and the improvement in survival grew increasingly larger throughout the first 10 years. The proportional reduction in mortality was similar in both node $(-)$ and node $(+)$ patients, but the absolute improvement in mortality reduction was greater in node $(+)$ women. In trials involving 5 years of tamoxifen, the absolute improvements in 10-year survival were 10.9% for node $(+)$ patients (61.4% vs 50.5%, $2p < 0.00001$) and 5.6% for node $(-)$ patients (78.9% vs 73.3%, $2p < 0.00001$). These benefits were noted regardless of age, menopausal status, tamoxifen dose, or whether chemotherapy was administered or not. Furthermore, the proportional reduction in contralateral breast cancer for 1 year, 2 years, and 5 years of tamoxifen use was 13%, 26%, and 47%, respectively. Thus, all patients with ER $(+)$ tumors should be considered for 5 years of adjuvant tamoxifen use.

Table 1
Five Years of Tamoxifen in the Overview

		ANNUAL % risk reductions:	
		Relapse	Death
Overall		42 ± 3	22 ± 4
Hormonal status	ER $\pm$	50 ± 4	28 ± 5
	ER unknown	37 ± 8	21 ± 9
	ER poor	6 ± 11	-3 ± 11
Lymphnodes	positive	43 ± 4	28 ± 6
	negative	49 ± 4	25 ± 5
Chemotherapy	C+T vs C	52 ± 8	47 ± 9
Dose	20 mg	45 ± 4	21 ± 6
	30–40 mg	49 ± 5	32 ± 6
Age	<50	45 ± 8	32 ± 10
	50–59	37 ± 6	11 ± 8
	60–69	54 ± 5	33 ± 6
	$\geqslant$70	54 ± 13	34 ± 13
	All ages	47 ± 3	26 ± 4

Outside of the overview, it is important to recognize the very large trials testing the newer selective aromatase inhibitors as adjuvant treatment for postmenopausal patients [14,15]. Together, these trials (ATAC and MA17) clearly show efficacy in terms of relapse-free survival for these agents. Whether they should be administered only after a course of tamoxifen (2 years? 5 years? Another duration?) or in place of tamoxifen remains highly uncertain.

Chemotherapy in the Overview

The activity of chemotherapy combined with the predictions of kinetic models of tumor growth and response to treatment led to the prediction that adjuvant therapy would be curative for some patients with early stage disease [16]. Following the first trials of adjuvant treatment, there have been hundreds of controlled and uncontrolled clinical trials designed to optimize therapy and identify specific approaches for selected subgroups of patients. The difficulty in interpreting this large body of data arises from the lack of consistent eligibility criteria, the sometimes subtle but potentially important variations in drug selection, dose, and schedule of administration among trials, as well as the generally modest impact of treatment. The latter point is critical because it renders phase II or pilot trials mostly uninterpretable and also makes small phase III trials potentially misleading. If the difference between two treatments is very small, then if by random chance a few more or less patients on one or the other arm of a trial experience a relapse or death, then the "true" benefit of a specific regimen may be obscured. To overcome this difficulty, the EBCTCG has performed three overviews (meta-analyses) of all available properly randomized systemic adjuvant therapy trials with more than five years of follow up beginning in 1985. The influential second overview was conducted in 1990 and published in 1992 [2] and the third conducted in 1995 and published in 1998 [3]. In evaluating these reports one must recognize both the strengths and weaknesses of the meta-analyses. Among these are the facts that the overview is a process of homogenization wherein similar, but not necessarily identical, trials are grouped together for analysis. For tamoxifen or ovarian ablation this is less of an issue as the treatments are by definition quite homogeneous but for chemotherapy it is a larger problem. Also, the overview is biased towards older trials because it requires at least 5 years of follow-up for inclusion, In addition it only provides indirect comparisons between treatment modalities, and is most powerful when examining very large groups and less so when attempting to identify relatively homogeneous treatment subgroups. In the latter circumstance, we lose power because the patient numbers become small. Another aspect of the overview is the method of reporting results. Both relative (proportional) odds reductions as well as absolute benefits (at fixed time points) are provided for each treatment modality and selected patient subgroups. The proportional benefits are always larger than the absolute ones, and application of these results to individual patients or groups of patients requires a sophisticated understanding of the difference between the two ways the benefits are reported along with a careful assessment of the underlying risk of recurrence.

For patients with hormone unresponsive tumors and those with high risk presentations, chemotherapy is a mainstay of treatment. However, the heterogeneity of systemic chemotherapy trials is far greater than that of the tamoxifen trials, making comparisons among the results of these studies even more difficult. As a result, the overview is somewhat less useful in guiding chemotherapy use than it is for tamoxifen. Included in the most recent overview were 47 trials with 18,000 patients randomly assigned to treatment versus none and about 6,000 each for trials of longer versus shorter durations of therapy and for regimens with or without anthracyclines [3]. Again, in contrast to the tamoxifen, a wide variation in the design of the specific regimens makes the conclusions of the meta-analysis less reliable and generalizable. If, for the sake of argument, one version of cyclophosphamide, methotrexate, and 5-fluorouracil (CMF) truly is superior to another, this will not be apparent in the overview where the many iterations of CMF are grouped together for analysis.

Table 2
Chemotherapy in the Overview

	Subgroups	ANNUAL % risk reductions	
		Relapse	Death
Age	All	23.8 ± 2.2	15.2 ± 2.4
	<40	37 ± 7	27 ± 8
	40–49	34 ± 5	27 ± 5
	50–59	22 ± 4	14 ± 4
	60–69	18 ± 4	8 ± 4
	70 and older	Uncertain	Uncertain
Regimen	CMF alone	24 ± 3	14 ± 4
	CMF plus other drugs	20 ± 5	15 ± 5
	Drugs other than CMF	25 ± 4	17 ± 4
	Anthracyclines vs CMF	12 ± 4	11 ± 5

Moreover, the potential impact of an "ideal" CMF will be obscured in this example. Hence, one must view the results of the chemotherapy overview with caution. In considering which regimen to use as standard therapy, oncologists should also note that the recent rapid evolution in the design of chemotherapy regimens involving potential improvements in dose, schedule, drug selection is not reflected in the overview. As a result, it is entirely possible that we may choose specific treatments which are not evaluated in the overview. In this case we view the overview as a means of confirming the principle that chemotherapy is effective even if we chose other specific regimens for use.

In women under the age of 50 years, prolonged polychemotherapy consisting of multiple agents administered over several months or longer decreased the annual risk of relapse by 35% and mortality by 27%. At 10 years of follow up, the absolute mortality reduction was 7% in patients with node-negative tumors and 11% in those with node-positive tumors [3]. (See Table 2) As with tamoxifen, the relative risk reductions for relapse rate and mortality were not significantly different for women with or without nodal involvement, but the absolute benefits were higher in women with lymph node involvement. For women over the age of 50 years, the benefits were somewhat smaller but still significant with annual risk reductions of 20% for recurrence and 11% for mortality seen. In this group the absolute gains in mortality after 10 years were 2% and 3% in node-negative versus node positive tumors, respectively.

DURATION OF CHEMOTHERAPY

Despite the attempt, as part of the overview, to define the optimal duration of therapy, it is probably unreasonable to expect a single answer to this question. Clearly, for each individual regimen there may be an optimal duration of therapy but the overview, since it consists of a heterogeneous group of such studies, is not the appropriate source for this answer. It is also possible that individual patients, based on their risk level and perhaps aspects of their tumor, might optimally benefit from differing durations of treatment.

For CMF and similar regimens, where the overview is strongest, treatment beyond 6 months does not improve either the mortality or relapse rates but a single treatment cycle was inferior to longer treatment regimens [3]. Hence, for CMF 6 months of treatment is an appropriate duration. For other regimens, such as doxorubicin and cyclophosphamide (AC), 3 months has been equivalent to 6 cycles of classical CMF and is therefore also appropriate [17] although longer durations of CAF may be slightly superior [18].

OTHER CHEMOTHERAPY REGIMENS

CMF is widely accepted as standard adjuvant therapy for lower risk patients. However, results from the overview and from individual studies suggest that other frequently used adjuvant regimens such as AC and 5-fluorouracil, doxorubicin, and cyclophosphamide (FAC) might be more active, possibly in selected subgroups. For example, in the overview about 6,000 patients were included from trials comparing CMF or similar regimens to anthracycline-containing treatments and a small, but significant, advantage for the latter was seen. The proportional risks for recurrence and mortality were reduced by 12% and 11%, and the absolute benefit was increased by 3.2% and 2.7%, respectively [3]. While small, note that these benefits are over and above those seen for CMF without the anthracycline. There are additional reasons to consider doxorubicin or epirubicin based regimens. The NSABP B15 trial compared 4 cycles of AC with 6 cycles of classical CMF and suggested that the shorter AC regimen was less toxic, mainly because it was half as long [17]. Efficacy in this trial was no different for the two regimens, but in several newer trials an advantage for the doxorubicin (or epirubicin) containing arm has been seen [18, 19]. One possibility, now being very carefully pursued, is that specific predictive factors can be used to identify subsets of patients who will benefit from the inclusion of anthracyclines. A recent example is the human epidermal growth factor receptor 2 (HER-2/neu). Preclinical experiments suggest that the introduction of additional copies of the HER-2/neu gene into cells growing in culture renders them more aggressive [20,21] but also more likely to require doxorubicin for treatment [22]. Several large retrospective studies are providing evidence that this may be true in the clinic as well [23–25]. If confirmed, HER-2/neu testing could become a critical step in determining the optimal chemotherapy regimen for specific patients. For example, among patients with node-negative disease, perhaps those with increased HER-2/neu gene number or receptor expression would be appropriate candidates for AC while perhaps those with HER-2/neu normal (negative) tumors could avoid potential long term cardiac toxicities by receiving CMF. Information on this possibility may be provided by re-analysis of the most recent report of a randomized trial (Intergroup INT 0102) directly comparing CMF and CAF in high risk node-negative patients with or without tamoxifen [18]. Because the overall differences in outcome on this study, while significant, are small, and given the special toxicities of the anthracyclines, clinicians can certainly use CMF routinely in low risk patients with node-negative disease. However, as described above, the emerging evidence concerning the interaction between HER-2/neu amplification and/or overexpression and doxorubicin use and dose may change this in the near future.

NEW DIRECTIONS IN CHEMOTHERAPY

Clinical research in recent years has focused on the use of dose-escalated therapy and the role of new active drugs, such as the taxanes. Despite pre-clinical models suggesting significant benefits to dose-escalation and intensity [26] as well as a great many promising phase II studies, a clear and consistent benefit for higher dose therapy has not been seen, especially when considering dose levels significantly above standard [27–33]. As a result high dose therapy remains investigational as discussed below. At the same time, we are beginning to get positive results from phase III trials testing taxanes and these results should influence standard practice [34, 35].

DOSE-ESCALATION

Laboratory evidence for a steep dose to response relationship, in particular for alkylating agents, has led to numerous feasibility and pilot trials utilizing autologous stem cells collected from the marrow or, more recently, peripherally, to support maximally escalated doses of chemotherapy. Because kinetic models of tumor growth and chemotherapy response suggested that the greatest likelihood for cure would be in the minimal tumor burden situation, patients with high risk early stage disease have been included in these studies. Promising non-randomized results have allowed high dose adjuvant chemotherapy to become very popular and it is frequently considered a standard treatment for high risk breast cancer. However, studies comparing conventional dose chemotherapy versus high-dose chemotherapy followed by stem cell transplant (HDCT/SCT) have mostly been negative in the adjuvant setting for high-risk node-positive patients [27–30]. A few trials suggest benefits for HDCT/SCT in subsets of patients. Roche et al showed an improvement in disease-free survival in those with 7–10 positive nodes [31]. Recently, Tallman et al showed a statistically significantly improved time to recurrence in those assigned to HDCT/SCT, who fulfilled strict eligibility criteria [32]. Rodenhuis et al. demonstrated improved relapse-free survival in those with 10 or more positive nodes and those with Her2/neu-normal tumors [33]. None of these trials showed overall survival (OS) benefit in all patients. Overall, results with dose escalation with HDCT/SCT have been mixed and efficacy has not been confirmed.

Taken together with the negative results available for dose escalation of cyclophosphamide above 600 mg/m^2 from the NSABP trials B22 and B25 [36,37] and the negative results for doxorubicin dose-escalation above 60 mg/m^2 in the recent CALGB trial (9344) [34], clinicians should remain cautious regarding the use of maximally dose-escalated therapy.

DOSE DENSE CHEMOTHERAPY REGIMENS

Dose-intensity is a way of quantifying the total amount of drug administered over a specified period of time. Increases in dose-intensity are therefore possible not only by increasing dose size (dose-escalation) but also by decreasing the interval between treatments (shortening the time period). The latter method for dose-intensification, first proposed by Norton and Simon, can be labeled "dose-dense" treatment to distinguish it from all other dose-intensification schemas [38]. A trial conducted in Milan and enrolling women with 4 or more involved nodes was one of the best tests of dose-dense therapy [39]. Here treatment consisted of alternating (less dose-dense) versus a sequential (more dose-dense) regimens using single agent doxorubicin (A) and CMF, and over 33 weeks of treat-

ment every patient on the study received 4 doses of doxorubicin and 8 of CMF. At 10 years of follow-up, sequential administration (4 cycles of A followed by 8 of CMF) remained significantly better in disease-free and overall survival than the alternating plan. Based on these results plus those of several promising pilot trials, the Intergroup has now conducted several trials where dose-density is a critical question. One study compared concurrent AC versus sequential (more dose-dense) administration of the same cumulative doses of these drugs (SWOG 9313). However, the numbers of cycles of administration for each agent vary in this trial. Coupled with the lack of a dose-response relationship in the super-normal range for these two drugs one has to recognize that rather than testing dose-density in isolation, this trial tests fewer cycles of higher dose treatment against more cycles of lower dose therapy. If the low and high doses are equally effective, this trial could be interpreted as showing that dose-dense administration of cyclophoshamide compensates for the administration of fewer cycles [40]. Another important trial compared every other week chemotherapy with every third week treatment (CALGB 9741) and demonstrated a significant improvement in both disease-free and overall survival for the more dose-dense approach [41]. (See Table 3).

Taxanes

In addition to improvements in dose and schedule of administration, another route to improved systemic treatment is the addition or substitution of new active agents to existing regimens. In this regard, one of the most significant developments in conventional chemotherapy in the past decade is the discovery of the efficacy, feasibility, and non-cross-resistance of the taxanes, including paclitaxel and docetaxel [42–44]. In advanced disease, paclitaxel is being extensively studied using a variety of doses and schedules but it is not yet certain which provides the optimal efficacy and toxicity profile. Docetaxel is also being tested over a more narrow range of doses and schedules. Because they are so active and apparently non-cross-resistant with doxorubicin, they have great potential in the adjuvant setting where some relapses may be presumed to be due to chemotherapy resistance. Several promising pilot trials established the feasibility of adding paclitaxel to escalated dose versions of either sequential or concurrent AC paving the way for large scale phase III testing [44].

Table 3
Ongoing/Planned Randomized Trials of Chemotherapy

Principle tested	Treatment	Study
High dose therapy	Cb followed by PSC or ABMT	NCI-G97-1145
	A → CMF vs A → CMF & HDCT	SCTN-BR9405, EU-95048
	CAF vs CAF & HDCT (closed 5/98)	CLB-9082, INT-0163, SWOG-9114
	CAF vs CAF & HDCT & PSC (closed 7/98)	EST-2190, INT-0121, SWOG-9061
	EC followed by SD CMF vs EC and HD EC	IBCSG-15-95, EU-96021
	ATC vs SD AC & PSC/ABMT	SWOG/Intergroup S9623
Dose dense therapy	AC vs A → C (closed 5/97)	SWOG 9313
	Sequential ATC vs AC?T q 14d vs q 21d	CLB-9741
	CMF vs Sequential E?CMF	SCTN-BR9601, EU-97013
	FAC vs FAC → CVP	CAN-OTT-9101
Neoadjuvant vs adjuvant	A → CMF vs AT → CMF vs AT → surgery → CMF	INT-23/96, EU-97001)
	Preop AC vs Preop AC → D vs Preop A then postop D	NSABP-B-27
	Preop vs Postop FEC x4	EORTC-10902
	Preop vs Postop FLAC	NCI-90-C-0044F,
	Neoadj FAC vs Neoadj CMF	GOCS-08-BR-95-III
Role of Herceptin[TM]	AC → T +/− H → Surgery → +/−H	CALGB proposed
	AC → T vs D → H	NCCTCG proposed
	AC → D with H	NSABP proposed

HDCT: High Dose Chemotherapy, SD: Standard Dose, PSC: peripher blood stem cell infusion, ABMT: autologous bone marrow transplant, E: Epirubicin, A: doxorubicin, C: cyclophosphamide, M: methotrexate, F: 5-fluorouracil, T: thiotepa, Cb: carboplatin, T: paclitaxel, L: Leucovorin, D: docetaxel, H: Herceptin[TM].

The first completed trial was the Cancer and Leukemia Group B study (9344) in which 3,170 women with involved axillary nodes were randomly assigned to treatment with AC (60/600 mg/m^2) alone or AC followed by four doses of paclitaxel (175 mg/m^2) over 3 hours every third week. All hormone receptor (HR) patients received adjuvant tamoxifen for 5 years. At 18 months median follow-up, there was a significant overall advantage for the addition of paclitaxel in both disease-free and overall survival [34]. The final publication at 69 months again showed a statistically significant difference in disease-free survival (DFS) and OS. With longer follow-up at 5 years, the hazard reductions from adding paclitaxel to AC were 17% for recurrence (DFS of 65% for AC alone vs 70% for AC → paclitaxel; $p = 0.0023$) and 18% for death (OS of 77% for AC and 80% for AC → paclitaxel; $p = 0.0064$). In a planned subset analysis defined by the protocol, the benefits of paclitaxel were similar regardless of tumor size, number of positive nodes, or menopausal status. The National Surgical Adjuvant Breast and Bowel Project (NSABP) B-28 was also conducted to compare the outcome of 3060 node-positive patients who received 4 cycles of AC (60/600 mg/m^2) followed by 4 cycles of paclitaxel (225 mg/m^2) versus no further chemotherapy [35]. Patients with HR-positive tumors received tamoxifen for 5 years, starting the first day of chemotherapy. The final results were reported recently at a median follow-up of 64 months with 861 events and 498 deaths. At 5 years the hazard reduction of recur-

rence for addition of paclitaxel was 17% (DFS of 72% for AC alone vs 76% for AC → paclitaxel; $p = 0.008$) and OS was 85% for both groups ($p = 0.46$). There was no significant interaction between treatment effect and HR status. Paclitaxel was beneficial regardless of age, tamoxifen administration, number of positive nodes, type of surgery, tumor grade, or histologic type. There were fewer deaths in AC → paclitaxel groups but no statistically significant impact is yet seen on survival. Of note, the patient population in CALGB 9344 was a higher risk group than those of NSABP B-28, and perhaps longer follow up may reveal delayed OS benefit with a lower risk population. Thus far, results of NSABP B-28, similar to CALGB 9344, support the use of paclitaxel following AC in node-positive breast cancer patients.

Another adjuvant trial, in which docetaxel replaced 5-fluorouracil as a component of a FAC regimen (FAC vs TAC) was recently updated and confirmed both a disease-free and overall survival advantage for the taxane-containing arm [45]. Combined with the promising results of several trials testing docetaxel in the pre-operative setting, it seems fair to conclude that both taxanes are active and appropriate candidates for standard use in the adjuvant setting.

A large number of studies that will address the relative value of the taxanes, the possible benefits of newer dose and schedule combinations (see Table 3) and the potential value of trastuzumab (Herceptin^{TM}) which is discussed below remain unreported to date.

RISK ASSESSMENT

The preceding discussion focused on the potential benefits of a variety of specific treatment options. However, a critical component of treatment decisions concerns the assessment of risk of relapse. Without this information it is not possible to determine the likely benefit of therapy for individual patients since, as described earlier, the relative risk reductions for treatment are constant but the absolute benefit changes with the level of underlying risk. At some low level of risk, many physicians and patients might conclude that the risks of a specific treatment might outweigh the potential benefits. To determine the risk or relapse (and death) in patients with invasive breast cancer, the most well-established prognostic factors are lymph node status and tumor diameter in that order. Histology is important, especially in patients with node negative disease, but most invasive tumors are of either of ductal or lobular type and the prognosis of these tumor types is similar.

Grade may distinguish higher and lower risk subsets in this setting. Patients with negative nodes and tumors of tubular, medullary or colloid type up to 2–3 cm have a more favorable prognosis than do those with ductal or lobular carcinoma of the same size [46]. Based on the risk of relapse seen following a median of 18 years follow-up of a large series of surgically treated patients with node-negative disease, those with invasive ductal or lobular histologies measuring up to 1 cm on microscopic examination have been considered candidates for observation while those with larger tumors deemed to have sufficient risk to warrant the potential toxicities of systemic therapy [47]. Of course any improvement in treatment such that the therapeutic index is increased, will serve to lower the threshold for treatment and increase the number of potential beneficiaries of adjuvant therapy.

In addition to the factors described above, there are a number of potentially useful markers of risk and also of response. The first example of the latter is the estrogen (and progesterone) receptor which identifies patients most likely to benefit from tamoxifen [5]. Although initially promising, other factors such as S-phase, ploidy, cathepsin-D have not been consistently useful on a routine basis and can be omitted from routine use [48]. Recently, however, HER-2/neu has been studied as it appears to be both prognostic and predictive [49,50]. Amplification of the gene and/or over-expression of the receptor is detected in 25–30% of breast cancers, depending in part on the specific test used as well as the def-

inition of overexpression. Despite the current heterogeneity of testing methods and results [51], HER-/neu status appears to correlate with prognosis, chemotherapy resistance in general, and sensitivity to moderately increased doses of doxorubicin [24,50]. In addition, in advanced disease those patients with tumors with high HER-2/neu overexpression were found to be more sensitive to taxanes when compared to tumors with low expression [52]. Studies are currently evaluating these correlations in the recent large adjuvant trials conducted within the intergroup. Pending the outcomes of these ongoing studies, using these various prognostic and predictive factors for clinical decision making can be challenging although the use of HER-2/neu status to select patients for doxorubicin-based adjuvant therapy is a reasonable approach [23–25]. Very recently, a novel test that integrates the results of an expression analysis that can be performed for a limited number of genes in paraffin embedded tissue, became available. Among tamoxifen-treated node-negative patients, this test appears to discriminate residual risk better than conventional approaches. Prospective studies are planned but for patients whose risk is less clear this test may be a useful tool in making the decision to offer or withhold chemotherapy [53].

THE NEXT STEP

The development of a recombinant humanized monoclonal antibody directed against the HER2/Neu protein (rhuMabHER2, trastuzumab,: Herceptin^{TM}) has been an exciting breakthrough in medical oncology. This is the first prospectively developed targeted agent since the advent of anti-estrogens and the first to interfere with the growth regulating HER2/neu influenced pathway. In addition to the evolving role of trastuzumab as treatment for breast cancer of all stages, this suggests that even better targeted therapies may be possible in the near future. Based particularly on the results of a pivotal multi-center trial of AC or paclitaxel with or without trastuzumab in patients with metastatic disease overexpressing HER-2neu [54], a series of adjuvant trials are now planned or beginning. Because of the increased risk of congestive heart failure seen in combination with doxorubicin [54], the adjuvant trials are all focusing on paclitaxel or docetaxel with or followed by trastuzumab. (See Table 3). These trials will be critical in establishing the safety and potential efficacy of this agent as adjuvant treatment in selected subgroups of patients.

In addition to new chemotherapy agents, it is possible that we will define a role for other established drugs as well. An example is the bisphosphonates which are already known to be effective in treating osteoporosis and in delaying the progression of lytic bone metastases [55]. Several intriguing European trials suggest that these agents may also offer adjuvant benefit [56,57] and large trials testing these agents are being planned.

For the new future it is also probable that anti-estrogens that are more selective in their effect than tamoxifen could play a role, not only in the adjuvant treatment of breast cancer, but also in prevention. The first of these, raloxifene, is now being compared to tamoxifen in a prevention trial [58] but other even more active agents may prove to be superior. Clinical trials testing specific SERMs as adjuvant treatment and prevention are already planned. Also in the early stages of development are anti-tumor vaccines, such as MUC-1 and STM, which are attractive non-toxic treatment and prevention alternatives, although efficacy data is not yet available. A polyvalent vaccine based on these and other antigens, such as VEG-F and HER-2/neu, is a current goal of laboratory and clinical studies.

CONCLUSION

Systemic adjuvant therapy, while a standard and proven component of the multi-modality care of women with breast cancer, continues to rapidly evolve. The most certain means of improving upon currently achievable outcomes is to consistently apply the most appropriate treatment options and to participate in clinical trials where possible. The specific approach to recommend for individual patients outside of clinical trials is best defined by the results of the overview and relevant randomized studies and varies with different clinical circumstances. In general, premenopausal patients are treated with chemotherapy if they have involved axillary nodes or invasive ductal or lobular carcinoma exceeding 1 centimeter in greatest diameter. Older women are treated similarly although with advancing years of life, the impact of chemotherapy appears to diminish, and in all patients comorbidities must be considered. All patients with positive HR assays are potential candidates for treatment with hormone therapy regardless of age and this treatment is additive to the benefits of chemotherapy [59]. A role for the aromatase inhibitors in post-menopausal patients is established but the best plan for incorporating them is not defined Specific chemotherapy options outside of clinical trials include CMF, AC, AC followed by paclitaxel, docetaxel concurrent with AC, as well as a variety of other anthracycline-containing regimens such as FEC or CEF. In general, lower risk patients can be treated with CMF while those with positive nodes can consider the anthracyclines and the taxanes. Clarification on the role of anthracylines in node-negative disease should be forthcoming, but it is very possible that patients with HER-2/neu positive tumors will benefit incrementally from the inclusion of an anthracycline. Novel dose and schedule strategies, such as dose-escalation and dose-dense treatments have been studied: the former are not effective but the latter is, Immunotherapy agents, such as the recombinant humanized monoclonal antibody against HER-2/neu and vaccines, should yield improved outcomes in selected subgroups of patients, but data from clinical trials will not be available for several years. Enrollment of eligible patients in these studies is one of our highest priorities.

REFERENCES

[1] Early Breast Cancer Trialists' Collaborative Group: Treatment of early breast cancer, vol. 1: worldwide evidence 1985–1990. Oxford?: Oxford University Press, 1990.

[2] Early Breast Cancer Trialists' Collaborative Group: Systematic treatment of early breast cancer by hormonal, cytotoxic, or immune therapy? 133 randomised trials involving 31,000 recurrences and 24,000 deaths among 75,000 women, *Lancet* **339** (1992), 1–15, 71–85.

[3] Early Breast Cancer Trialists' Collaborative Group: Polychemotherapy for early breast cancer: an overview f the randomized trials, *Lancet* **352** (1998), 930–942.

[4] Early Breast Cancer Trialists' Collaborative Group: Analysis overview results. Presented at the Fifth Meeting of the Early Breast Cancer Trialists Collaborative Group, Oxford, United Kingdom, September 21–23, 2000 abstract.

[5] Tamoxifen for early breast cancer: an overview of the randomised trials, Early Breast Cancer Trialists' Collaborative Group, *Lancet* **351** (1998), 1451–1467.

[6] Ovarian ablation in early breast cancer: overview of the randomized trials. Early Breast Cancer Trialists' Collaborative Group, *Lancet* **348** (1996), 1189–1196.

[7] W.A. Woodward, E.A. Strom, S.L. Tucker et al., Changes in the 2003 American Joint Committee on Cancer Staging for breast cancer dramatically affect stage-specific survival, *J Clin Oncol* **21** (2003), 3244–3248.

[8] F. Cardoso, Microarray technology and its effect on breast cancer classification and prediction of outcome, *Breast Cancer Res* **5** (2003), 303–304.

[9] S.H. Giordano, A.U. Buzdar, T.L. Smith et al., Is breast cancer survival improving? *Cancer* **100** (2004), 44–52.

[10] G.T. Beatson, On the treatment of inoperable cases of carcinoma of the mamma: suggestions for a new method of treatment, with illustrative cases, *Lancet* **ii** (1896), 104–107.

[11] F. Boccardo, A. Rubagotti, D. Amoroso et al., Cyclophosphamide, methotrexate, and fluorouracil versus tamoxifen

plus ovarian suppression as adjuvant treatment of estrogen receptor-positive pre-/perimenopausal breast cancer patients: results of the Italian Breast Cancer Adjuvant Study Group 02 randomized trial, *J Clin Oncol* **18** (2000), 2718–2727.

[12] P. Schmid, M. Untch, D. Wallwiener et al., Cyclophosphamide, methotrexate and fluorouracil (CMF) versus hormonal ablation with leuprolide acetate as adjuvant treatment of node-positive, premenopausal breast cancer patients: preliminary results of the TABLE-study (Takeda Adjuvant Breast cancer study with Leuprolide Acetate), *Anticancer Res* **22** (2002), 2325–2332.

[13] R. Jakesz, H. Hausmaninger and H. Samonigg, Chemotherapy versus hormonal adjuvant treatment in premenopausal patients with breast cancer, *Eur J Cancer* **38** (2002), 327–332.

[14] M. Baum, A.U. Buzdar, J. Cuzick et al., Anastrozole alone or in combination with tamoxifen versus tamoxifen alone for adjuvant treatment of postmenopausal women with early breast cancer: first results of the ATAC randomized trial, *Lancet* **359** (2002), 2131–2139.

[15] P.E. Goss, J.N. Ingle, S. Martino et al., A randomized trial of letrozole in postmenopausal women after five years of tamoxifen therapy for early-stage breast cancer, *N Engl J Med* **349** (2003), 1793–1802.

[16] H.E. Skipper, Kinetics of mammary tumor cell growth and implications for therapy, *Cancer* **28** (1971), 1479–1499.

[17] B. Fisher, A.M. Brown, N.V. Dimitrov, R. Poisson et al., Two months of doxorubicin-cyclophosphamide with and without interval reinduction therapy compared with 6 months of cyclophosphamide, methotrexate, and fluorouracil in positive-node breast cancer patients with tamoxifen-nonresponsive tumors: Results from the National Surgical Adjuvant Breast and Bowel Project B-15, *J Clin Oncol* **8** (1990), 1483–1496.

[18] L. Hutchins, S. Green, P. Ravdin, D. Lew, S. Martino, M. Abeloff, A. Lyss, C. Henderson, C. Allred, S. Dakhil, I. Pierce, W. Goodwin, J. Caton, S. Rivkin, R. Chapman and K. Osborne, CMF versus CAF with and without tamoxifen in high-risk node-negative breast cancer patients and a natural history follow-up study in low-risk node-negative patients: first results of intergroup trial INT 0102, *Proc Am Soc Clin Oncol* **17**(1a) (1998), (abstr 2).

[19] M.N. Levine, V.H. Bramwell, K.I. Pritchard et al., Randomized trial of intensive cyclophosphamide, epirubicin, and fluorouracil chemotherapy compared with cyclophosphamide, methotrexate and fluorouracil in premenopausal women with node-positive breast cancer, *J Clin Oncol* **16**(8) (1998), 2651–2658.

[20] P.P. DiFiore, J.H. Pierce, H.J. Kraus et al., erb B-2 is a potent oncogene when overexpressed in NIH-3T3 cells, *Science* **237** (1987), 178–182.

[21] R.M. Hudziak, J. Schlessinger and A. Ullrich, Increased expression of the putative growth factor receptor p185HER causes transformation and tumorigenesis of NIH-3T3 cells, *Proc Natl Acad Sci USA* **84** (1987), 7159–7163.

[22] M. Campiglio, G. Somenzi, C. Olgiati et al., Role of proliferation in HER2 status predicted response to doxorubicin, *Int J Cancer* **105** (2003), 568–573.

[23] S. Paik, J. Bryant, C. Park et al., erb B-2 and response to doxorubicin in patients with axillary lymph node-positive, hormone receptor-negative breast cancer, *J Natl Cancer Inst* **90** (1998), 1361–1370.

[24] A.D. Thor, D.A. Berry, D.R. Budman et al., erbB-2, p-53, and efficacy of adjuvant therapy in lymph node-positive breast cancer, *J Natl Cancer Inst* **90** (1998), 1346–1360.

[25] A. Moliterni, S. Menard, P. Valagussa et al., HER2 overexpression and doxorubicin in adjuvant chemotherapy for resectable breast cancer, *J Clin Oncol* **21** (2003), 458–462.

[26] D.D. Von Hoff, G.M. Clark, G.R. Weiss et al., Use of in vitro dose-response effect to select antineoplastics for high-dose or regional administration regimens, *J Clin Oncol* **4** (1986), 1827–1834.

[27] The Scandinavian Breast Cancer Study Group 9401. Results from a randomised adjuvant breast cancer study with high dose chemotherapy with CTCb supported by autologous bone marrow stem cells versus dose escalated and tailored FEC therapy, *Proc Am Soc Clin Oncol* **18**(2a) (1999), (abstr).

[28] G.N. Hortobagyi, A.U. Buzdar, R.L. Theriault et al., Randomized trial of high-dose chemotherapy and blood cell autografts for high-risk primary breast carcinoma, *J Natl Cancer Inst* **92** (2000), 225–233.

[29] W.P. Peters, G. Rosner, J. Vredenburgh et al., Updated results of a prospective, randomized comparison of two doses of combination alkylating agents (AA) as consolidation after CAF in high-risk primary breast cancer involving ten or more axillary lymph nodes (LN): CALGB 9082/SWOG 9114/NCIC Ma-13, *Proc Am Soc Clin Oncol* **20**(21a) (2001), (abstr 81).

[30] J.P. Crown, M. Lind, A. Gould et al., High-dose chemotherapy (HDC) with autograft (PBP) support is not superior to cyclophosphamide (CPA), methotrexate and 5-FU (CMF) following doxorubicin (D) induction in patients (pts) with breast cancer (BC) and 4 or more involved axillary lymph nodes (4+LN): The Anglo-Celtic I study, *Proc Am Soc Clin Oncol* **21**(42a) (2002), (abstr 166).

[31] H.H. Roche, P. Pouillart, N. Meyer et al., Adjuvant high dose chemotherapy (HDC) improves early outcome for high risk (>7) breast cancer patients: the Pegase 01 trial, *Proc Am Soc Clin Oncol* **20**(26a) (2001), (abstr).

[32] M.S. Tallman, R. Gray, N.J. Robert et al., Conventional adjuvant chemotherapy with or without high-dose chemotherapy and autologous stem-cell transplantation in high-risk breast cancer, *N Engl J Med* **349** (2003), 17–26.

[33] S. Rodenhuis, M. Bontenbal, L. Beex et al., High-dose chemotherapy with hematopoetic stem-cell rescue for high-risk breast cancer, *N Engl J Med* **349** (2003), 7–16.

[34] I.C. Henderson, D.A. Berry, G.D. Demetri et al., Improved outcomes from adding sequential paclitaxel but not from escalating doxorubicin dose in an adjuvant chemotherapy regimen for patients with node-positive primary breast cancer, *J Clin Oncol* **21** (2003), 976–983.

[35] E.P. Mamounas, J. Bryant, B.C. Lembersky et al., Paclitaxel (T) following doxorubicin/cyclophosphamide (AC) as adjuvant chemotherapy for node-positive breast cancer: results from NSABP-B 28, *Proc Am Soc Clin Oncol* **22**(4a) (2003), (abstr 12).

[36] B. Fisher, S. Anderson, D.L. Wickerham et al., Increased intensification and total dose of cyclophosphamide in a doxorubicin-cyclophosphamide regimen for the treatment of primary breast cancer: findings from National Surgical Adjuvant Breast and Bowel Project B-22, *J Clin Oncol* **15** (1997), 1858–1869.

[37] B. Fisher, S. Anderson, A. DeCillis et al., Further evaluation of intensified and increased total dose of cyclophosphamide for the treatment of primary breast cancer: Findings from National Surgical Adjuvant Breast and Bowel Project B-25, *J Clin Oncol* **17** (1999), 3374–3388.

[38] L. Norton and R. Simon, Tumor size, sensitivity to therapy, and design of treatment schedules, *Cancer Treat Rep* **61** (1977), 1307–1317.

[39] G. Bonadonna, M. Zambette and P. Valagussa, Sequential or alternating doxorubicin and CMF regimens in breast cancer with more than three positive nodes, *JAMA* **273** (1995), 542–547.

[40] C. Haskell, S. Green, G. Sledge et al., Phase III comparison of adjuvant high-dose doxorubicin plus cyclophosphamide (AC) versus sequential doxorubicin followed by cyclophosphamide (A->C) in breast cancer patients with 0–3 positive nodes (intergroup 0137), *Proc. Am Soc. Clin. Onc* **21** (2002), p. abstract 142.

[41] M.L. Citron, D.A. Berry, C. Cirrincione et al., Randomized trial of dose-dense versus conventionally scheduled and sequential versus concurrent combination chemotherapy as postoperative adjuvant treatment of node-positive primary breast cancer: first report of Intergroup Trial C9741/Cancer and Leukemia Group B Trial 9741, *J Clin Oncol* **21** (2003), 1431–1439.

[42] C. Bernard-Marty, F. Cardoso and M.J. Piccart, Use and abuse of taxanes in the management of metastatic breast cancer, *Eur J Cancer* **39** (2003), 1978–1989.

[43] M. Levin, The role of taxanes in breast cancer treatment, *Drugs Today* **37** (2001), 57–65.

[44] C. Hudis, Adjuvant use of taxanes for patients with breast cancer: we see the tip of the iceberg, *Clin Breast Cancer* **3** (2002), 326–332.

[45] M. Martin, T. Pienkowski, J. Mackey et al., TAC improves disease free survival and overall survival over FAC in node positive early breast cancer patients, BCIRG 001: 55 months follow-up, *San Antonio Breast Cancer Symposium* (2003), (abstr 43).

[46] G.N. Hortobagyi, Treatment of breast cancer, *N Engl J Med* **339** (1998), 974–984.

[47] P.P. Rosen, S. Groshen, P.E. Saigo et al., Pathologic prognostic factors in stage I (T1N0M0) and stage II (T1N1M0) breast carcinoma: a study of 644 patients with median follow-up of 18 years, *J Clin Oncol* **7** (1989), 1239–1251.

[48] E.G. Mansour, P.M. Ravdin and L. Dressler, Prognostic factors in early breast carcinoma, *Cancer* **74** (1994), 381–400.

[49] D.J. Slamon, G.M. Clark, S.G. Wong, W.J. Levin, A. Ullrich and W.L. McGuire, Human breast cancer: correlation of relapse and survival with amplification of the HER-2/neu oncogene, *Science* **235** (1987), 177–182.

[50] M.D. Pegram, G.Pauletti and D.J. Slamon, HER-2/neu as a predictive marker of response to breast cancer therapy, *Breast Cancer Res Treat* **51** (1998), 65–77.

[51] M. Fornier, M. Risio, Van Poznak et al., HER2 testing and correlation with efficacy of trastuzumab therapy, *Oncology* **16** (2003), 1340–1348, 1351–1352.

[52] J. Baselga, A.D. Seidman, P.P. Rosen et al., HER2 overexpression and paclitaxel sensitivity in breast cancer therapeutic implications, *Oncology* **11** (1997), 43–48.

[53] S. Paik, S. Shak, G. Tang et al., Multi-gene RT-PCR assay for predicting recurrence in node-negative breast cancer patients: NSABP studies B-20 and B-14, *San Antonio Breast Cancer Symposium* (2003), (abstr 16).

[54] D.J. Slamon, B. Leyland-Jones, S. Shak et al., Use of chemotherapy plus a monoclonal antibody against HER2 for metastatic breast cancer that overexpresses HER2, *N Engl J Med* **344** (2001), 783–792.

[55] I.J. Diel, E.F. Solomayer and G. Bastert, Treatment of metastatic bone disease in breast cancer, *Clin Breast Cancer* **1** (2000), 43–51.

[56] I.J. Diel, E.F. Solomayer, S.D. Costa et al., Reduction in new metastases in breast cancer with adjuvant clodronate treatment, *N Engl J Med* **339** (1998), 357–363.

[57] T. Powles, S. Paterson, J.A. Kanis et al., Randomized, placebo-controlled trial of clodronate in patients with primary operable breast cancer, *J Clin Oncol* **20**, 3219–3224.

[58] B.K. Dunn and L.G. Ford, From adjuvant therapy to breast cancer prevention: BCPT and STAR, *Breast J* **7** (2001), 144–157.

[59] B. Fisher, J. Dignam, N. Wolmark et al., Tamoxifen and chemotherapy for lymph node-negative, estrogen receptor-positive breast cancer, *J Natl Cancer Inst* **89** (1997), 1673–1682.

Breast Disease 21 (2004) 15–21
IOS Press

Management Recommendations for Adjuvant Systemic Breast Cancer Therapy

Edith A. Perez*
Multidisciplinary Breast Clinic and Division of Hematology/Oncology, Mayo Clinic and Mayo Foundation, Jacksonville, FL, USA

Keywords: Adjuvant therapy, breast cancer, anti-estrogens, chemotherapy

INTRODUCTION

It is estimated that over 211,000 women in the United States will be diagnosed with breast cancer in the year 2003 [1]. Despite the modest decreases in the age-adjusted mortality rate for breast cancer that have occurred since the 1980's, methods to further improve these rates are needed. Appropriate local therapy remains the cornerstone of treatment for patients with non-metastatic breast cancer. Methods to achieve this goal include earlier diagnosis, better general medical care, and appropriate administration of systemic adjuvant treatments following resection of breast cancer. A large amount of data have been accumulated over the last few years, helping us to better understand the utilization of ovarian ablation, hormonal therapy, and chemotherapy, as well as local treatments for patients with early breast cancer. Some of these data were discussed as part of the Early Breast Cancer Trialists' Group (EBCTG) conferences in 1998 and 2000 [2,3], the 2000 National Institutes of Health (NIH) Consensus Conference [4], and the St. Gallen meetings from 2001 and 2003 [5].

Several important trials evaluating ovarian ablation, aromatase inhibitors, taxanes, and schedule of chemotherapy are relevant to clinical practice. Systemic chemotherapy, with or without hormonal therapy based on the biological characteristics of the tumor, is the current standard of treatment for patients with node-positive breast cancer, and for a large portion of those with node-negative disease and invasive tumors measuring >1.0 cm. Ultimately, the success of adjuvant therapy will depend not only on optimizing current regimens, but also on exploring new therapeutic targets, improving the understanding of individual tumor and patient characteristics that influence treatment selection and outcome, critical analysis and integration of data, consensus building, and education regarding the results of these analyses.

Ongoing studies increasingly incorporate recently obtained knowledge of the biology of breast cancer, and incorporate targeted approaches. But even before new data are generated, the overall results from the studies already reported are consistent with significant improvements in disease-free and overall survival for all groups of patients: pre- or postmenopausal, node positive or negative breast cancer.

HORMONAL THERAPY

Ovarian ablation has been found to lead to fairly similar outcomes compared to older chemotherapy regimens, such as cyclophosphamide, methotrexate and fluorouracil (CMF), for premenopausal women [6,7]. The role of ovarian ablation in combination with chemotherapy remains a matter for further study. Trials to

---

*Address/reprint requests: Edith A. Perez, MD, Professor of Medicine, Division of Hematology and Oncology, Mayo Clinic, 4500 San Pablo Road, Jacksonville, FL 32224, USA. Tel.: +1 904 953 7283; Fax: +1 904 953 6178; E-mail: perez.edith@ mayo.edu.

better evaluate ovarian ablation in premenopausal patients who have not received chemotherapy or those who remain premenopausal after receiving systemic chemotherapy are under way (Fig. 1). They include the SOFT, TEXT, and PERCHE trials, amongst others. The 3 main studies eluded to are a result of worldwide collaboration between different breast cancer cooperative groups. There is a clear consensus that tamoxifen should not be recommended for patients with estrogen receptor-negative breast cancer (either for prevention of recurrence or prophylaxis for contralateral breast cancer. This recommendation is supported not only by the EBCTG meta-analyses, but specifically by data from the National Surgical Adjuvant Breast and Bowel Project (NSABP) B-23 and the Intergroup study INT102 [8,9]. These two studies not only failed to demonstrate benefit for tamoxifen in patients with estrogen receptor-negative breast cancer, but also did not demonstrate that tamoxifen decreased contralateral breast cancer in patients with primary estrogen receptor-negative disease. The presence or absence of HER2 expression should not be a determinant of whether to use hormonal therapy, based on currently available data.

Five years of tamoxifen has been recommended for patients with measured >1.0 cm, independent of menopausal state or lymph node status [4]. This was based on large amounts of data, including the findings from the EBCTG demonstrating a highly statistically significant 47% reduction in annual odds of recurrence and a 26% reduction in annual odds of death for patients with estrogen receptor-positive tumors receiving 5 years of tamoxifen.

The role of aromatase inhibitors instead of tamoxifen for postmenopausal patients is becoming increasingly important in view of the data from the anastrozole, tamoxifen, alone or in combination (ATAC) trial [10, 11]. The ATAC study demonstrated a small, but statistically significant, improvement in disease-free survival for postmenopausal patients with resected breast cancer who received anastrozole instead of tamoxifen, but not for the concurrent use of tamoxifen with anastrozole [10,11].

CHEMOTHERAPY

Advances in adjuvant chemotherapy for the treatment of women with early-stage breast cancer have generally been incremental. In the 1970s, cyclophosphamide, methotrexate, fluorouracil (CMF) was the gold standard, while in the 1980s, data began to emerge demonstrating the effectiveness of anthracyclines in the adjuvant setting. In the 1990s, anthracyclines became the mainstay of adjuvant chemotherapy, largely because of the Early Breast Cancer Trialists' Collaborative Group overview analysis [2]. Indeed, in the 1995 review of poly-chemotherapy for early breast cancer, which compared with standard CMF alone, as well as anthracycline-containing regimens with CMF as adjuvant therapy, it was shown that compared with standard CMF alone, anthracycline-containing regimens reduced the annual risk of breast cancer recurrence by 12%, and the annual risk of death by 11% [2]. Findings from the 2000 overview analysis confirm these findings. As such, current worldwide consensus statements and recommendations on the treatment of early breast cancer suggest anthracycline-containing regimens be used as adjuvant therapy for most women with early-stage disease [3–5].

The EBCTG meta-analysis published in 1998, after review of adjuvant therapy trials that started before 1990, reported that chemotherapy reduced the annual odds of recurrence by 40% in patients younger than 50 years of age with estrogen receptor-negative tumors and by 33% in those with estrogen receptor-positive disease [3]. This apparent difference, based on receptor status, was not statistically significant. Similarly, there was a 30% reduction in the annual odds of recurrence in patients older than 50 with estrogen receptor-negative tumors and an 18% reduction in those with estrogen receptor-positive tumors.

The 2000 NIH Consensus Conference addressed several issues regarding chemotherapy worthy of mention [4]. It was recommended that the majority of women should receive systemic chemotherapy for four to six courses. Randomized trials of the same chemotherapy given four or six times have not been completed, so it was difficult to issue a definite statement regarding the exact number of months or cycles for which chemotherapy should be given.

Adjuvant anthracycline polychemotherapy continues to have a meaningful, though modest, impact on the outcome of women with early-stage breast cancer. The optimal anthracycline-containing adjuvant chemotherapy regimen remains the subject of debate. Chemotherapy dose, dose-intensity, duration of treatment, schedule, and toxicities should be considered in therapeutic decisions. Randomized trials have demonstrated that four cycles of anthracycline-containing regimens consisting of two drugs are, at best, equivalent to CMF in terms of relapse-free and overall survival rates, while six or more cycles of anthracycline-containing regimens consisting of three or more drugs have demonstrated superiority [2–4,9,10,13,14]. Indeed, ongoing trials will give us definitive answers.

The taxanes, which are also very active agents, are under intense investigation in the adjuvant setting to determine if further incremental benefit can be gained. The use of taxanes was not strongly recommended in the Consensus meetings in the years 2000 and 2001, partly due to the short follow-up of the few studies available at the time [4,15]. However, new data have emerged since then and will be reviewed in the next sections. Patient and tumor characteristics for the adjuvant taxane studies reported so far are described in Table 1.

To date, efficacy results from various randomized trials evaluating adjuvant taxanes have been reported: three with paclitaxel and one with docetaxel (Table 2, Table 3). One of the paclitaxel trials, a US Intergroup trial (CALBG 9344), evaluated sequential paclitaxel following various anthracycline-containing regimen doxorubicin/ cyclophosphamide [AC], demonstrating a statistically significant improvement in disease-free and overall survival with the addition of paclitaxel, but no difference based on the dose of doxorubicin used [16]. A second recently reported trial of the US Intergroup (CALBG 9741), was a phase III 2:2 randomized trial comparing dose-dense (every 2 weeks with growth factor support) versus conventional (every 3 weeks) scheduling, and sequential versus concurrent administration. At a median follow-up time of 34 months, this study demonstrated significant improvements in disease-free and overall survival with dose-dense chemotherapy, over conventional dosing (Table 2, Table 3) [19]. This improvement using a more frequent chemotherapy schedule was accompanied by generally better tolerability (except for anemia and increased blood transfusions), but was accompanied by a significant increase in cost due to the need for growth factor support with all cycles of treatment.

BCIRG 001: First Planned Interim Analysis

The first planned interim analysis of the BCIRG 001 trial, after a median follow-up of 33 months, has demonstrated a statistically significant 8% absolute improvement in the primary endpoint of disease-free survival with TAC, compared with FAC (82% vs. 74%, $P = 0.0011$) [18]. This improvement in disease-free survival was independent of hormone receptor status because both estrogen receptor- positive and –negative

patients clearly benefited from TAC. Importantly, the duration of therapy was similar between the taxane and non-taxane arms (>90% of patients in each group received the six scheduled cycles), eliminating the potential influence of this parameter on the survival outcomes. At this point of median follow-up, no statistically significant difference is evident in overall survival between the two groups, with TAC conferring an absolute 5% advantage in this secondary endpoint, compared with FAC (92% vs. 87%, $P = 0.11$). Conversely, in the subset of patients with one to three positive nodes, overall survival was significantly higher in those randomized to TAC rather that FAC (96% vs. 89%, $P = 0.006$).

In terms of tolerability, TAC was associated with a 24% incidence of febrile neutropenia (despite the use of prophylactic ciprofloxacin), compared with a 2% incidence in the FAC group. At the same time, however, there were no between-group differences in sepsis or deaths from infectious complications (no septic deaths were reported in either group). The incidence of grade 3 and 4 infection was 3% in the TAC group and 1.5% in the FAC group. TAC was also associated with a rate of asthenia twice that of FAC, with incidences of 11% and 5%, respectively, in BCIRG 001. Although this increased incidence of asthenia is noteworthy, it is a short-term rather than a long-term complication.

Of the docetaxel trials with adequate follow-up, interim results of the Breast Cancer International Research Group 001 trial demonstrated that substituting docetaxel for fluorouracil in combination with doxorubicin and cyclophosphamide (TAC) resulted in improved disease-free survival regardless of hormone receptor status, with a trend toward improved overall survival [18]. The significant increased risk of febrile neutropenia observed with the TAC regimen utilized, essentially mandates the use of growth factor support [19].

National Surgical Adjuvant Breast and Bowel Project (NSABP) B-28

Cancer and Leukemia Group B (CALBG) Intergroup 9344 and National Surgical Adjuvant Breast and Bowel Project (NSABP) B-28 [16,17]. Both of these trials evaluated a sequential approach with doxorubicin and cyclophosphamide (AC) followed by single-agent paclitaxel in patients with node-positive breast cancer. In CALBG 9344, 3170 patients were randomly assigned to receive either doxorubicin, 60, 75, or 90 mg/m^2 plus cyclophosphamide, 600 mg/m^2 every 3 weeks

Table 1
Reported Taxane Adjuvant Trials: Patient and tumor characteristics

	Intergroup CALBG 9344 [16]	NSABP B-28 [17]	BCIRG 001 [18]	Intergroup C9741 [19]
Patients, n	3170	3060	1491	2005
Age <50 years	60	51	54	60
Lymph node involvement				
1–3 nodes	46	70	62	59
>4 nodes	54	30	38	41
T >2 cm	63	41	60	60
ER and/or PR positive	65	66	69	65
Tamoxifen use	60	84	69	69

BCIRG – Breast Cancer International Research Group; CALBG-Cancer and Leukemia Group B; ER-estrogen receptor; NSABP- National Surgical Adjuvant Breast and Bowel Project; PR-progesterone receptor; T-tumor

Table 2
Relative reduction in risk of relapse in taxanes adjuvant trials

	Intergroup CALBG 9344 [16]	NSABP B-28 NIH 11/00 [17]	BCIRG 001 NIH 11/00 [18]	Intergroup C9741 [19]
Median follow-up, mo	69	34	33	34
Relapse risk reduction, %	18	7	32	26
Hazard ratio	0.88	0.93	0.68	0.74
	(0.77–1.00)	(0.78–1.10)	(0.54–0.86)	
	$P = 0.0324$	$P = 0.38$	$P = 0.0011$	$P = 0.010$

ASCO-American Society of Clinical Oncology; BCIRG-Breast Cancer International Research Group; CALBG-Cancer and Leukemia Group B; mo=months; NIH-National Institutes of Health

for four cycles followed by paclitaxel, 175 mg/m^2 every 3 weeks for four cycles, or no further chemotherapy [16]. NSABP B-28 had a similar design, with 3060 node-positive patients receiving four cycles of standard AC (doxorubicin, 60 mg/m^2 plus cyclophosphamide, 600 mg/m^2 every 3 weeks) followed by four cycles of paclitaxel, 225 mg/m^2 every 3 weeks, or no further chemotherapy [17].

Studies are ongoing to address how best to incorporate the taxanes into therapy: in place of the anthracycline, in combination with the anthracycline, or in sequence with an anthracycline (CTSU website: www.ctsu.org). To date, it is clear that the addition of a taxane does indeed provide further benefit with respect to relapse rates and in some studies also survival and represents a valuable component of adjuvant chemotherapy for patients with node-positive breast cancer, including those with estrogen receptor positivity and/or extensive lymph node involvement. Further data are needed regarding the role of taxanes in patients with node-negative disease.

Another way to evaluate the benefits of adjuvant taxane therapy is to review the absolute differences in disease-free and overall survival. As shown in Table 3, the absolute disease-free survival benefits for taxane therapy in CALGB 9344 and BCIRG 001 were 6% and 8%, respectively; corresponding improvements in overall survival were 6% and 5%, respectively. Both the C9741 Intergroup and BCIRG 001 trial demonstrate similar absolute benefits in disease-free and overall survival.

TARGETED THERAPIES

An exciting area of research is the incorporation of targeted treatments in the adjuvant setting [4,5,21, 22]. However, none are ready for general use at this time. The only targeted therapy approved for use in the metastatic setting, other than anti-estrogens, is trastuzumab, an agent that is now being evaluated in four well-planned worldwide adjuvant trials conducted by cooperative groups [22,23]. Completion of recruitment and analysis of the data demonstrating a benefit of this anti-HER2 monoclonal antibody when added to chemotherapy could be a major advance in the treatment of patients at high risk of relapse following resection of invasive breast cancer. Additionally, all of these studies include the prospective collection of tumor specimens, which will assist in the understanding of the biology of breast cancer [24].

Consensus Conferences, Clinical Trials, Actual use of Adjuvant Chemotherapy

In spite of the demonstrated efficacy of adjuvant chemotherapy in prolonging survival for women with invasive breast cancer, and management recommenda-

Table 3
Absolute Disease-free and overall survival absolute differences reported in taxane adjuvant trial

	Intergroup CALBG 9344 (69-months) [16]			NSABP B-28 (34-months) [17]			BCIRG 001 (33-months) follow-up [18]			Intergroup C9741 (34-months) [19]		
	AC + P	AC	Difference %	AC→P	AC	Difference %	TAC	FAC	Difference %	Q 2W	Q 3W	Difference %
DFS, %	79	75	5*				82	74	8*	82	75	7*
OS, %	88	85	3*				92	87	5	92	90	2*

*=statistically significant.

Table 4
Adjuvant Chemotherapy: Impact of the Addition of a Taxane

Therapy	Sample size	Follow-up	Recurrence reduction in annual odds, %	Death reduction in annual odds, %
Anthracycline vs. no anthracycline [2,4]	∼7,000	15 yr	23.5	17
Paclitaxel vs. no paclitaxel [5,14]	∼3,000	69 mo	17	18
Docetaxel vs. no docetaxel [17]	1,491	33 mo	32	24*

*= not significant.

tions by consensus panels, many patients are not receiving these treatments. This may be most pronounced in women as they age. First of all, a report from Hutchins and colleagues highlighted that only 9% of the patients enrolled in breast cancer trials were 65 years or older [25]. This is in the setting of this group accounting for approximately 40% of patients diagnosed with this disease. The barriers for this disparity regarding accrual to clinical trials are multi-factional, and one of the most important may be physician bias regarding the benefit or tolerability of older women to the currently available agents [26,27].

Moreover, many of those patients may only be offered CMF chemotherapy due to a perception of it being less toxic. There are several problems with this thinking including the following: 1) if "classic" CMF is utilized (which in a randomized clinical trial has been demonstrated to be superior to intravenous once every three week CMF), only 60% of patients are able to receive the six intended doses of therapy due to toxicity; 2) six cycles of adjuvant CMF have been demonstrated to be less efficacious to six-cycles of anthracycline-based chemotherapy [2,4,9,10]; 3) older women have been shown to tolerate chemotherapy in a fairly similar way as younger women (if end-organ function and performance status are not impaired) [27,28].

The Intergroup CALBG 49907 trial described earlier in this manuscript is bringing attention to this issue. Additionally, the recent meta-analysis demonstrating that older women derive as much benefit from systemic adjuvant chemotherapy compared to younger women will be critically important to be disseminated amongst not only physicians but also allied health staff and patients [29].

A recent report by Du and colleagues addresses the discrepancy between Consensus recommendations and actual community use of systemic chemotherapy [30]. These investigators performed a cohort study of 5101 women 20 years of age or older diagnosed with stages I-IIIA breast cancer in New Mexico from 1991–1997. The evaluation consisted of pattern of chemotherapy by age and demonstrated that 29% of women received this systemic treatment (11% Stage I, 47% Stage II, and 68% Stage IIIA). They also found that the use of chemotherapy decreased substantially with increasing age. Overall, 18% of women ages 60–64 received chemotherapy, versus 31% of those ages 55–59, 44% of those between ages 50–54 and 66% of women younger than 45 years of age. An important potential implication is that many unnecessary deaths may be occurring due to the lack of application of guidelines (such as the NIH 2000 Consensus Conference recommending adjuvant chemotherapy for premenopausal or postmenopausal women with node-positive tumors or node-negative tumors of >1 cm, regardless of hormone status). One of the conclusions from this study was that outcome studies should address whether recommendations from consensus panels are overly aggressive or whether practicing oncologists are just too conservative in their use of chemotherapy.

CONCLUSIONS

Selection of optimal adjuvant systemic therapy for breast cancer patients with resected breast cancer is a challenging undertaking. It requires translating data from clinical trials that have involved thousands of patients into a highly individualized, risk-adjusted approach. Choosing adjuvant therapy for women with breast cancer requires consideration of four factors: A) evaluation of risk of relapse; B) extrapolation of results from clinical trials; C) therapeutic ratio, and D) the patient's preferences following a thorough discussion with her physician. Data from recently completed phase III adjuvant trials and worldwide consensus conferences document the benefits of adjuvant therapy in improving disease-free survival and overall survival for patients diagnosed with invasive breast cancer >1.0 cm in size. The benefits of hormonal therapy are clear, but limited to patients with estrogen receptor-positive breast cancer. Data with tamoxifen indicate that this agent should be used sequentially with chemotherapy [31].

Anthracyclines lead to improved outcomes compared with non-anthracycline regimens. Some studies of taxanes demonstrated that these agents improve disease-free survival and overall survival in patients with node-positive disease. Ongoing studies expanding investigation of biological predictors of outcome and response, and integrating targeted therapies with optimal chemotherapy schedules, should continue advancing the field and yielding improved outcomes for patients eligible to receive adjuvant therapies for breast cancer.

REFERENCES

[1] A. Jemal, T. Murray, A. Samuels, A. Ghafoor, E. Ward and M. Thun, Cancer Statistics, 2003, *CA Cancer J Clin* **53** (2003), 5–6.

[2] Early Breast Cancer Trialists' Collaborative Group (EBCTCG). Polychemotherapy for early breast cancer: an overview of the randomized trials, *Lancet* **352**(9132) (1998), 930–942.

[3] Early Breast Cancer Trialists' Collaborative Group (EBCTCG). Tamoxifen for early breast cancer: an overview of the randomized trials, *Lancet* **351**(9114) (1998), 1451–1467.

[4] National Institutes of Health Consensus Development. National Institutes of Health Consensus Development Conference Statement: Adjuvant therapy for breast cancer, November 1–3, 2000, *J Natl Cancer Inst* **93**(13) (2001), 979–989.

[5] A. Goldhirsch, J.H. Glick, R.D. Gelber and H.J. Senn, Meeting highlights: International Consensus Panel on the Treatment of Primary Breast Cancer, *J Natl Cancer Inst* **90**(21) (1998), 1601–1608.

[6] W. Jonat, M. Kaufmann, R. Sauerbrei et al., Goserelin Versus Cyclophosphamide, Methotrexate, and Fluorouracil as Adjuvant Therapy in Premenopausal Patients with Node-Positive Breast Cancer: The Zoladex Early Breast Cancer Research Association Study, *J Clin Oncol* **20**(24) (2002), 4628–4635.

[7] R. Jakesz, H. Hausmaninger, E. Kubista et al., Randomized Adjuvant Trial of Tamoxifen and Goserelin Versus Cyclophosphamide, Methotrexate , and Fluorouracil: Evidence for the Superiority of Treatment with Endocrine Blockade in Premenopausal Patients with Hormone-Responsive Breast Cancer – Austrian Breast and Colorectal Cancer Study Group Trial 5, *J Clin Oncol* **20**(24) (2002), 4621–4627.

[8] B. Fisher, S. Anderson, E. Tan-Chiu, N. Wolmark et al., Tamoxifen and Chemotherapy for Axillary Node-Negative, Estrogen Receptor-Negative Breast Cancer: Findings from National Surgical Adjuvant Breast and Bowel Project B-23, *J Clin Oncol* **19**(4) (2001), 931–942.

[9] L. Hutchins, S. Green, P. Ravdin et al., CMF versus CAF with and without tamoxifen in high-risk node-negative breast cancer patients and a natural history follow-up study in low-risk node-negative patients: first results of Intergroup trial INT 0102, *Proc Am Soc Clin Oncol* **17** (1998), 1a.

[10] K.I. Pritchard, M.N. Levine, V.H.C. Bramwell et al., A randomized trial comparing CEF to CMF in premenopausal women with node positive breast cancer: update of NCIC CTG MA.5. SABCS 2002.

[11] The ATAC (Arimidex, Tamoxifen Alone or in Combination Trialists Group) Anastrozole alone or in combination with tamoxifen versus tamoxifen alone for adjuvant treatment of postmenopausal women with early breast cancer: first results of the ATAC randomized trial, *Lancet* **359**(9324) (2002), 2131–2139.

[12] The ATAC (Arimidex, Tamoxifen Alone or in Combination Trialists Group) Pharmacokinetics of anastrozole and tamoxifen alone, and in combination, during adjuvant endocrine therapy for early breast cancer in postmenopausal women: a sub-protocol of the Arimidex and Tamoxifen Alone or in Combination (ATAC) trial, *Br J Cancer* **85**(3) (2001), 317–324.

[13] R. Peto, EBCTGG: Updated results from September 2000 worldwide overview, *Eur J Cancer* **36**(Suppl 5) (2000), 847.

[14] B.A. Mincey, F.M. Palmieri and E.A. Perez, Adjuvant Therapy for Breast Cancer: Recommendations for Management Based on Consensus Review and Recent Clinical Trials, *The Oncologist* **7** (2002), 246–250.

[15] E.A. Perez, Incorporation of Taxanes in the Adjuvant Management of Patients with Breast Cancer: 2000 NIH Consensus Development Conference, *Advances in Breast Cancer* **3**(2) (2001), 2–5.

[16] C.I. Henderson, D.A. Berry, G.D. Demetri et al., Improved Outcomes from Adding Sequential Paclitaxel but not From Escalating Doxorubicin Dose in an Adjuvant Chemotherapy Regimen for Patients with Node-positive Primary Breast Cancer, *J Clin Oncol* (2003), in press.

[17] E.P. Mamounas, J. Bryant, B.C. Lembersky et al., Paclitaxel (T) following doxorubicin/cyclophosphamide (AC) as adjuvant chemotherapy for node-positive breast cancer: Results from NSABP B-28. ASCO 2003, abstract #12.

[18] J.M. Nabholtz, J. Pienkowski, M. Mackey et al., Phase III trial comparing TAC (docetaxel, doxorubicin, cyclophosphamide) with FAC (5-fluorouracil, doxorubicin, cyclophosphamide) in the adjuvant treatment of node positive breast cancer (BC) patients: interim analysis of the BCIRG001 study, *Proc Am Soc Clin Oncol* **21**(1) (2002), 36a.

[19] M.L. Citron, D.A. Berry, C. Cirrincione et al., Randomized trial of dose-dense versus conventionally scheduled and sequential versus concurrent combination chemotherapy as postoperative adjuvant treatment of node-positive primary breast cancer: first report of Intergroup Trial C9741/Cancer and Leukemia Group B Trial 9741, *J Clin Oncol* **21**(7) (2003), in press.

[20] E.A. Perez, Adjuvant Therapy Approaches to Breast Cancer: Should Taxanes be Incorporated? *Curr Oncol Rep* **5** (2003), 66–71.

[21] E.A. Perez, HER-2 as a Prognostic, Predictive, and Therapeutic Target in Breast Cancer, *Cancer Control* **6**(3) (1999), 233–240.

[22] E.A. Perez, Adjuvant anti-HER2 monoclonal antibody therapy – ready for breast cancer? *The Breast* **10**(Suppl 3) (2001), 161–163.

[23] E.A. Perez, Phase III trial of doxorubicin and cyclophosphamide (AC) followed by weekly paclitaxel with or without trastuzumab as adjuvant treatment for patients with HER2 overexpressing or amplified node positive breast cancer. (N9831) (IRB 1770-1799). www.

[24] E.A. Perez, P.C. Roche, R.C. Jenkins, C.R. Reynolds, K.C. Halling, J.N. Ingle and L.E. Wold, HER2 testing in breast cancer. Poor correlation between weak positivity by Immunohistochemistry (2^+) and gene amplification by fluorescence in situ hybridization, *Mayo Clin Proc* **77** (2002), 148–154.

[25] L.F. Hutchins, J.M. Unger, J.J. Crowley, C.A. Coltman and K.S. Albain, Under-representation of patients 65 years or older in cancer-treatment trials, *N Engl J Med* **341** (1999), 2061–2067. (PMID: 10615079).

[26] H.B. Muss, The role of chemotherapy and adjuvant therapy in the management of breast cancer in older women, *Cancer* **74** (1994), 2165–2171. (PMID: 11773294).

[27] H.B. Muss, Chemotherapy of breast cancer in older patients, *Semin Oncol* **22** (1995), 14–16. (PMID: 7863346).

[28] E.A. Perez, C.L. Vogel, D.H. Irwin, J.J. Kirshner and R. Patel, Weekly Paclitaxel in Women Age 65 and above with Metastatic Breast Cancer, *Breast Cancer Res and Treat* **73**(1) (2002), 85–88.

[29] H.B. Muss, S.H. Woolf, D.A. Berry et al., Older women with node positive (N^+) breast cancer (BC) get similar benefits from adjuvant chemotherapy (Adj) as younger patients (pts): The Cancer and Leukemia Group B (CALBG) experience. ASCO 2003, abstract #11.

[30] X.L. Du, C.R. Key, C. Osborne, J.D. Mahken and J.S. Goodwin, Discrepancy between Consensus Recommendations and actual community use of adjuvant chemotherapy in women with breast cancer, *Ann Intern Med* **138** (2003), 90–97.

[31] K.S. Albain, S.J. Green, P.M. Ravdin, C.D. Bobau, E.G. Levine, J.N. Ingle et al., Adjuvant chemohormonal therapy for primary breast cancer should be sequential instead of concurrent; initial results from Intergroup trial 0100 (SWOG-5814), *Proc Am Soc Clin Oncol* **21**(1) (2002), 37a.

Breast Disease 21 (2004) 23–31
IOS Press

Neoadjuvant Chemotherapy

Marjorie C. Green*, Francisco J. Esteva and Gabriel N. Hortobagyi
University of Texas M.D. Anderson Cancer Center, Houston, TX, USA

Keywords: Neoadjuvant chemotherapy, breast cancer

BACKGROUND

While the incidence of breast cancer is rising, mortality is actually declining [1]. This decline in mortality may be due to multiple factors including earlier stage of disease at diagnosis, improved local therapy techniques and also improvements in the medical management of breast cancer. It has been well demonstrated that the use of endocrine therapy and/or systemic chemotherapy improves survival for all subsets of patients with curable breast cancer, both in individual trials as well as in recent meta-analyses [2,3]. Despite the advances that have been made, many women will still unfortunately develop fatal recurrences of their breast cancer. Without therapy, even patients with stage I breast cancer have a greater than 10% risk of recurrence over a 5–10 year period [4]. Treatment with systemic chemotherapy and/or endocrine therapy can reduce but not eliminate the risk of recurrence. It is believed that for these patients who develop recurrence, micrometastatic disease is present at the time of diagnosis and that systemic therapy was unable to eradicate malignant cells. Different treatment approaches have been designed to help improve overall survival including the recent practice of using non- cross-resistant therapies as treatments of curable breast cancer [5–7] One treatment approach that continues to undergo evaluation is the use of neoadjuvant chemotherapy.

There are multiple potential advantages to the use of neoadjuvant chemotherapy. Preclinical data suggests that the removal of the primary tumor can lead to accelerated growth of micrometastatic disease [8]. Administration of chemotherapy prior to the removal of the primary tumor may therefore help to eliminate any micrometastatic disease prior to a potential growth spurt experienced after surgery. The use of cyclophosphamide in mice as treatment of implanted mammary tumors was found in one study to be most effective when given prior to the removal of the largest tumor giving credence to this hypothesis [9]. These studies helped to spark interest in the use of neoadjuvant chemotherapy as a treatment approach that could potentially improve survival. It has also been suggested that delivery of chemotherapy as soon as possible after diagnosis will be helpful in that fewer micrometastases will be established therefore improving the odds that therapy will work [10].

Experience with neoadjuvant chemotherapy for locally advanced breast cancer had shown several other appreciable benefits for this treatment approach. The use of neoadjuvant chemotherapy for patients with stage IIIA- IIIB breast cancer has been well described [11]. Chemotherapy given in the neoadjuvant setting for inoperable breast cancer allows many patients to successfully undergo local therapy. Up to 80% of patients treated with chemotherapy or endocrine therapy have objective responses and a small percentage of these patients will have a complete response. This approach, applied to patients with earlier stages of breast cancer, could potentially offer improved rates of breast conservation. One of the potential disadvantages of administering systemic therapy prior to surgery is the loss of information regarding the number

---

*Corresponding author: Marjorie C. Green, M.D., Assistant Professor of Medicine, Breast Medical Oncology, The University of Texas M. D. Anderson Cancer Center, Box 424, 1515 Holcombe Blvd., Houston, TX 77030, USA. Tel.: +1 713 792 2817; Fax: +1 713 794 4385; E-mail: mgreen@mdanderson.org.

of axillary lymph nodes involved. However, in patients with locally advanced breast cancer the node status retains its prognostic significance following neoadjuvant chemotherapy [12]. Another attractive feature of this treatment approach is the ability to test the in vivo response to neoadjuvant chemotherapy. In the adjuvant setting, there are no definite markers to predict response to chemotherapy and it is uncertain which patients benefit from treatment. By administering the chemotherapy in the neoadjuvant setting, ineffective therapy can be withheld for patients who have primary resistance to therapy, thereby limiting the exposure to potentially toxic agents.

RANDOMIZED TRIALS

There are multiple phase II trials that demonstrate the potential of neoadjuvant chemotherapy for operable breast cancer yet only 8 completed randomized trials that evaluate the use of neoadjuvant chemotherapy directly compared with surgical resection followed by adjuvant therapy (Table 1). The primary endpoint for most of these trials is determination of the impact that the timing of chemotherapy has upon overall survival. The trials have differing periods of follow-up and definitions of response making direct comparisons between trials difficult.

The first study reported by Scholl in 1994 and updated by Broet in 1999 [13,14] randomized 390 premenopausal patients with stage I-IIIA (T2-3, N0) breast cancer to receive either four cycles of chemotherapy with doxorubicin, cyclophosphamide and 5-flurouracil followed by surgery or initial local therapy followed by chemotherapy with the same regimen. For this trial, local therapy for the adjuvant arm was considered to be radiation with or without surgery. Patients randomized to the adjuvant chemotherapy arm underwent radiation and if any residual disease was detectable after therapy, surgery with either segmental mastectomy or mastectomy was preformed. With this approach, 77% of patients had breast-conserving therapy (BCT), not significantly different when compared with an 82% rate of BCT for patients treated on the neoadjuvant arm. Initial reports described an improved 5 year overall survival for patients receiving neoadjuvant chemotherapy (86% vs. 78%, $p = 0.04$) however with longer follow-up the survival advantage of neoadjuvant chemotherapy (64.6%) over adjuvant therapy (60.2%) was no longer seen. (ref above)

The second study reported in 1994 compared the combination of radiation therapy and neoadjuvant chemotherapy versus radiation alone prior to surgery. All patients received 4–6 cycles of chemotherapy in the adjuvant setting allowing comparison of the timing of chemotherapy between treatment groups. In this study, 271 patients with stage IIB-IIIA breast cancer were randomized to receive either primary radiation or radiation combined with thiotepa, methotrexate and 5-fluorouracil. After completion of this treatment, all patients underwent modified radical mastectomy followed by an additional four to six cycles of chemotherapy. The patients receiving combined modality neoadjuvant chemotherapy had superior clinical response (12.4%) and pathologic response in the breast (29.1%) compared with those receiving only radiation therapy (5.9% and 19.4% respectively). Despite the improvement in clinical and pathologic response, no improvement in overall survival was seen between treatment arms [15].

A study published by Mauriac, et al. in 1999 [16] randomized patients with stage II-IIIA breast cancer to receive epirubicin, mitomycin C, thiotepa, and vindesine in either the neoadjuvant or adjuvant setting. Local therapy for these patients was guided by the timing of their therapy and clinical response. Patients in the adjuvant arm all underwent mastectomy whereas 69.9% of patients who received neoadjuvant therapy underwent breast-conserving therapy (BCT). Of patients undergoing BCT, 33% had primary irradiation of the breast without any surgical therapy. This study was initially reported with 34-month median follow-up. With additional time, it was found that 47% of patients who received primary irradiation as their only modality of treatment had a recurrence. The overall rate of BCT for the neoadjuvant arm therefore decreased to 45% at 124 months median follow-up. Of note, despite the increased risk of local recurrence for patients who underwent primary irradiation to the breast, there were no differences in overall survival between treatment groups and the local recurrence rate was very similar for patients who had surgical BCT (15%) vs. mastectomy (14%).

In 1997, Ragaz et al. reported a study evaluating one cycle of preoperative CMF followed by surgery and eight cycles of adjuvant CMF vs. the administration of nine cycles of CMF given entirely in the adjuvant setting for patients with stage I-II breast cancer [17]. With median follow-up of 10 years, no difference in overall survival was seen between treatment groups however it is uncertain what impact one cycle of chemother-

Table 1
Randomized Clinical Trials Evaluating Neoadjuvant Chemotherapy for Operable Breast Cancer

Reference:	Treatment	Clinical response rate	Pathologic response rate	OS
Broet (1999) [14]	CTX->XRT +/− Surgery (neoadjuvant) vs. XRT +/− Surgery –> CTX (adjuvant)	Neoadjuvant CTX: 65% (clinical CR) Primary XRT/ Adjuvant CXT: 85% (clinical CR)	———	Neoadjuvant: 64.6% (10-year) Adjuvant: 60.2% (10-year)
Semiglazov (1994) [15]	CTX + XRT –>Surgery–> CTX (neoadjuvant) vs. XRT–> Surgery–> CTX (adjuvant)	———	Neoadjuvant: 29.1% Adjuvant 19.4%	Neoadjuvant: 86.1% (5-year) Adjuvant: 78.3% (5-year) $p = ns$
Mauriac (1999) [16]	CTX–> XRT +/− Surgery (ncoadjuvant) vs. Surgery–> CTX (adjuvant)	Neoadjuvant: 33%	———	$p = ns$ (results not provided OS 55% at 10 years)
Ragaz (1997) [17]	CTX (one cycle)–> Surgery–> CTX (neoadjuvant) vs. Surgery–> CTX (adjuvant)	———	———	Neoadjuvant: 74% (10-year) Vs. Adjuvant: 73% (10-year) $p = ns$
Jakesz (2001) [18]	CTX –> Surgery –> CTX (neoadjuvant) vs. Surgery –> CTX (adjuvant)	———	Neoadjuvant: 6.0%	$P = NS$ (results not provided)
Makris (1998) [19]	CTX (+ Tam) –> Surgery (neoadjuvant) vs. Surgery–> CTX (+TAM)	Neoadjuvant: 32%		$p = ns$ (results not provided OS 78-80% at 4 years)
van der Hage (2001) [20]	CTX –> Surgery (neoadjuvant) vs. Surgery –> CTX (adjuvant)	Neoadjuvant: 6.6%	Neoadjuvant 4.28%	Neoadjuvant: 82% (4-years) Adjuvant: 84% (4-years) $p = ns$
Wolmark (2001) [21]	CTX–> Surgery (neoadjuvant) vs. Surgery–> CTX (adjuvant)	Neoadjuvant: 36%	Neoadjuvant: 13%	Neoadjuvant: 69% (9-year) Adjuvant: 70% (9-year) $p = ns$

CTX= chemotherapy.

apy given in the preoperative setting would make, recognizing that approximately 3 cycles of chemotherapy is needed to obtain a clinical PR. This study does show however that it is safe to administer a portion of chemotherapy to patients while they are waiting for surgery with no detriment in outcome.

A study presented at the American Society of Clinical Society (ASCO) annual meeting in 2001 by Jakesz et al. randomized patients with high-risk ER negative tumors (node- positive or large tumor size) to receive either neoadjuvant or adjuvant chemotherapy [18] All patients in the neoadjuvant arm received three cycles of CMF followed by surgery. Subsequent chemotherapy in the adjuvant setting was determined by nodal status. Patients with residual lymph node positive disease after neoadjuvant chemotherapy received three cycles of epirubicin and cyclophosphamide. Those patients with node- negative disease after neoadjuvant chemotherapy received three additional cycles of CMF. Patients treated in the adjuvant setting received sim-

ilar chemotherapy based upon nodal status. Because of the study design, the chemotherapy regimens were not balanced between treatment arms- there was a possibility that patients with lymph node positive disease in the neoadjuvant setting may have not received anthracycline-containing chemotherapy in the adjuvant setting. This could potentially decrease any survival advantage that otherwise would be seen for the neoadjuvant arm had all patients been treated based upon initial nodal status. Despite this potential bias, this study confirmed that neoadjuvant chemotherapy improved the rate of breast conserving therapy from 59.5% (adjuvant patients) to 66.7%. There was no statistically significant difference in disease-free or overall survival between treatment arms. Of note, patients who did not initially respond to neoadjuvant CMF had a statistically inferior disease free survival (48.1%) compared with those patients who had a response (70.8%) to the same regimen.

Makris et al. published updated data in 1998 of a study conducted in the early 1990's [19]. In this study, patients received neoadjuvant chemo/endocrine therapy with mitoxantrone and methotrexate $(+/-$ with mitomycin C) combined with tamoxifen for four cycles followed by four cycles of the same regimen in the adjuvant setting or they received eight cycles of chemo/endocrine therapy in the adjuvant setting. Patients in the neoadjuvant treatment group experienced an overall clinical response rate of 83% with a significant improvement in the rate of BCT compared to the adjuvant treatment group. As with the majority of randomized trials, with long term follow-up, no difference in DFS or OS was seen based upon the timing of therapy.

Two contemporary studies have evaluated neoadjuvant chemotherapy versus adjuvant chemotherapy with anthracycline containing regimens. The European Organization for Research and Treatment of Cancer (EORTC) conducted a study where patients with operable breast cancer received 5-fluorouracil, epirubicin and cyclophosphamide (FEC) in either the neoadjuvant or adjuvant settings [20]. With a median follow up of 56 months, patients receiving neoadjuvant therapy had similar DFS (65%) and OS (82%) compared with patients receiving adjuvant therapy (DFS- 70%, OS- 84%). (p – ns). There were also no differences in the local/regional recurrence rates between treatment groups.

The National Surgical Adjuvant Breast and Bowel Project (NSABP) B-18 compared the use of 4 cycles of neoadjuvant AC (60 mg/m2 doxorubicin/600 mg/m2 cyclophosphamide) compared with 4 cycles of AC given in the adjuvant setting for patients with stage I-IIIA breast cancer. In this study, patients were well matched between arms for tumor size, age and clinical nodal status. As with the majority of randomized studies, this trial examined the impact of the timing of chemotherapy on disease- free and overall survival [21, 22]. With a median follow-up of 5 years, there was no difference seen in DFS or OS (neoadjuvant: 72.3% vs. adjuvant: 73.2%) between treatment groups.

Even though there was no apparent survival difference observed in NSABP B-18 based purely on the timing of chemotherapy, several important observations were made. The use of neoadjuvant AC for four cycles allowed a higher rate of breast conserving therapy (67%) than seen for evenly matched patients who received adjuvant therapy (60%). As seen from the experience with locally advanced breast cancer, this difference was greatest for patients whose tumors were initially greater than 5.1 cm. Even with the improved rate of breast conservation, there was no statistically significant difference in local recurrence rates between treatment groups, i.e. the ability to improve breast conservation did not place the neoadjuvant patients at higher risk for local recurrence compared with patients treated in the adjuvant setting. Another important observation made during this study was based upon the clinical and pathologic complete response (pCR) obtained with neoadjuvant chemotherapy. The authors found that response could predict survival. Previous data published by the University of Texas M. D. Anderson Cancer Center for patients with locally advanced breast cancer linked clinical response to neoadjuvant chemotherapy with survival [23]. Similar data has also been described by Bonnadonna, et al. [24]. Evaluation of response from NSABP B-18 showed that patients who achieved a clinical CR after four cycles of neoadjuvant AC had a superior OS $(p = 0.0001)$ and DFS $(p = 0.0014)$ compared with patients who achieved a PR or less. Pathologic complete response (absence of invasive tumor in the breast) was even more specific- patients with a pCR had an overall survival rate of 88.7% – superior to all other groups who received therapy and still had residual disease at the time of surgery. $(p = 0.0004)$.

NEWER STUDIES REDEFINE THE ROLE OF NEOADJUVANT CHEMOTHERAPY

From the randomized trials it can be concluded that the timing of chemotherapy does not apparently impact upon survival. However, observations from these studies include: 1) breast conservation is enhanced with neoadjuvant chemotherapy; 2). local recurrence is not higher with this treatment approach; and 3) survival is not harmed by this strategy which make this an attractive treatment option for our patients. The finding that pCR predicts survival allows this treatment approach to be used to identify therapies that may likely improve survival without the need for long-term follow-up, thereby allowing implementation of effective therapies earlier in their clinical development. This feature of neoadjuvant therapy has influenced the design of many recent and ongoing trials investigating the role of taxanes as treatment for early-stage breast cancer. The definition of pCR varies widely however and attention should be focused upon the definition applied for clinical trials. For example, NSABP B-18 defines pCR as the absence of invasive tumor based upon serial sectioning of the breast without including data from lymph node evaluation. Other research groups combine data obtained from the breast and lymph nodes in their definition. The taxanes, paclitaxel and docetaxel have shown impressive activity against metastatic breast cancer [25] They offer a non-cross-resistant method of cytotoxic action against cancer cells when compared with the activity of anthracyclines making the taxanes an ideal complement to commonly used regimens (FEC, FAC, CAF, AC). Several studies in the adjuvant setting have shown that the addition of taxanes to anthracycline based treatment improves survival for early stage breast cancer. Data in the neoadjuvant setting also suggests that the use of these agents may impact upon the natural history of breast cancer.

One of the first studies presented that evaluates the use of neoadjuvant taxanes was published by Buzdar et al. in 1999 [26]. In this study patients with stage I-IIIA breast cancer were randomized to receive four cycles of FAC (500 mg/m2 5-fluorouracil/ 50 mg/m2 doxorubicin/ 500 mg/m2 cyclophosphamide) or four cycles of paclitaxel (225 mg/m2 given as a continuous infusion over 24 hours). After completion of chemotherapy, all patients underwent local treatment followed by an additional four cycles of FAC in the adjuvant setting. Evaluation of pCR found no statistical difference between FAC and paclitaxel. When these patients were analyzed with patients who received the same regimens in the adjuvant setting, patients who received four cycles of paclitaxel followed by four cycles of FAC had a trend towards superior DFS (86% at 48 months) compared with patients who received eight cycles of FAC (83%) ($p = 0.09$) [27]. A study presented by Green, et al. in 2002 compared the effect of differing schedules of taxanes upon the pCR for patients with operable breast cancer. As compared with NSABP B-18, in this study, pCR was defined as the absence of invasive tumor in the breast and axillary lymph nodes [28]. 258 patients with stage I-IIIA breast cancer were randomized to receive paclitaxel on either a weekly or q 3 week basis for 12 weeks followed by four cycles of FAC. The dose of paclitaxel in the weekly schedule varied based upon nodal status. Patients who had axillary lymph node involvement as confirmed by FNA of suspicious nodes (ultrasound) received a higher dose of paclitaxel (150 mg/m2/week) than those patients without abnormal appearing lymph nodes (80 mg/m2/week). Patients receiving paclitaxel on an every three-week schedule received this medication at a dose of 225 mg/m2 given as an infusion over 24 hours. All chemotherapy was administered in the neoadjuvant setting. Patients who received weekly paclitaxel followed by FAC ($n = 131$)

had a pCR in the breast and axillae of 28% compared with a pCR rate of 15% for patients who received q 3-week paclitaxel followed by FAC. Of note, the pCR rates were equivalent for the differing doses of weekly paclitaxel possibly suggesting that it is the schedule of paclitaxel that influenced the pCR rate rather than the dose of medication.

NSABP B-27 evaluated the sequential use of docetaxel after anthracycline- containing therapy for patients with operable breast cancer. 2411 patients with stage I-IIIA breast cancer were randomized to one of three groups. Group one received AC for four cycles followed by surgery. Group II received AC for four cycles and then docetaxel for four cycles followed by surgery. Group III received AC for four cycles followed by surgery followed by adjuvant docetaxel for four cycles. Presented at the San Antonio Breast Cancer Symposium in 2001, data from the AC neoadjuvant treatment groups (group I and III) was compared with the group receiving both AC and docetaxel (group II) in the neoadjuvant setting [29]. Patients receiving sequential therapy with AC followed by docetaxel had superior CR (65%) and pCR (25.6%- breast only) compared with patients receiving AC alone (CR-40%, pCR- 13.7%). In addition, patients receiving both treatments (AC, docetaxel) had improved pCR in the axilla (59.5%) compared with patients receiving AC alone (51.5%).

In addition to possibly identifying superior chemotherapy regimens earlier, the responses seen with differing regimens could also be used to predict the need for additional therapy/change to differing regimens. Two studies have been published where the response obtained with one regimen in the neoadjuvant setting determined subsequent therapy. The first study published by Smith et al. evaluated 162 patients with stage II- IIIB breast cancer who initially received CVAP (cyclophosphamide, vincristine, doxorubicine and prednisolone) for four cycles followed by evaluation for clinical response [30]. Patients who achieved a clinical CR or PR ($n = 104$) were randomized to receive additional therapy with CVAP or non-cross-resistant therapy with docetaxel for an additional four cycles. Patients who did not respond to therapy (stable disease or progression; $n = 55$) were switched without randomization to docetaxel. Of the patients who initially responded and then were maintained on CVAP, 18% had a pCR in the breast. Patients who had an initial response to CVAP and then were switched to docetaxel had a pCR of 34%. Based upon an intention-to-treat analysis, there was no statistical difference in pCR between the treatment arms ($p = 0.06$). Patients who did not initially respond to therapy and were subsequently switched to docetaxel had a low pCR of 2%. The improvement in pCR for the initial responders is reflected in DFS and OS. Those patients responding to CVAP who were maintained on the same regimen had a 3-year DFS of 71% and OS of 84% compared with patients who initially responded to CVAP and then were subsequently switched to docetaxel (DFS- 90% $p = 0.03$, OS- 97%; $p = 0.05$). In addition, the sequential use of CVAP–> docetaxel in responders was associated with a high rate of breast conserving therapy (67%) compared with responding patients who received only CVAP (48%).

The second study, from the University of Texas M. D. Anderson Cancer Center, evaluated patients with locally advanced breast cancer. Patients with stage IIIA and IIIB breast cancer received neoadjuvant VACP (vincristine, doxorubicin, cyclophosphamide and prednisone) for three cycles followed by local therapy. Patients who had residual disease in their breast after an initial response were randomized to receive either additional treatments with VACP or a different regimen (VbMF- vinblastine, methotrexate, 5-flourouracil) [31]. Those patients who had residual disease after VACP and were switched to receive VbMF had a trend towards higher DFS than those patients who were maintained on their initial therapy (46% vs. 25%, $p = 0.13$ at 125 months median follow-up). This study suggests that alteration of a therapeutic plan based upon response can possibly enhance survival. The ability to evaluate the in vivo response to chemotherapy can be used to tailor chemotherapy and possibly change outcome.

In general, approximately 5–10% of patients who would not have been candidates for breast conserving therapy become candidates after receiving neoadjuvant therapy. As seen with the experience with locally advanced breast cancer, this offers a clinically desirable endpoint for many patients. For patients who would never be breast conserving therapy candidates, the use of neoadjuvant chemotherapy is still a reasonable option. From the randomized trials presented it can be safely stated that neoadjuvant chemotherapy is a reasonable option for patients with early stage/operable breast cancer. There is no difference or detriment in overall survival from this treatment approach and when response to therapy is utilized to choose/tailor chemotherapy regimens, survival could possibly be improved.

Unanswered Questions

There are however several theoretical and occasionally practical problems when implementing the use of neoadjuvant chemotherapy for early-stage breast cancer into clinical practice. Evaluation of response to therapy is imperfect- whether based upon physical examination, radiographic studies or a combination of the two. For example, in NSABP B-27, 40% of patients who received AC for four cycles in the neoadjuvant setting achieved a clinical CR. Of these patients, only 13.7% achieved a pCR. Imaging modalities that could better predict pCR could help clinicians to modify therapy to avoid ineffective therapies and maximize response. Potential applications include positron emission tomography (PET) [32] or MRI [33] For example, in one study, researchers found that MRI accurately correlated tumor size with residual disease seen on pathologic samples for patients treated with neoadjuvant chemotherapy [34]. The use of these radiographic studies in correlation with clinical evaluation could help to modify the treatment plan for patients in real time.

In addition, there is some concern that local recurrence will be higher for patients who are treated with neoadjuvant therapy and that this difference could impact negatively upon survival. For example, in the EORTC study 10902 evaluating neoadjuvant FEC vs. adjuvant FEC, patients who were initially planned to undergo mastectomy but were "downstaged" so that BCT could be performed, were found to have decreased survival compared with patients who were initially planned to undergo BCT (HR 2.53, 95% CI 1.02–6.25). Despite this, there were no overall differences between local recurrence rates based upon the timing of therapy (neoadjuvant vs. adjuvant) or differences in survival seen between the randomized treatment arms. It is uncertain if this reported decline in survival is a true reflection of risk associated with neoadjuvant chemotherapy or possibly an artifact of an unplanned analysis. That is, it is unknown if the groups compared for this result were similar in their pretreatment characteristics (one assumes that the initial tumor size differs), the pCR to therapy (higher rate of residual disease in the group who converted to BCT could predict worsened survival) and the local therapy delivered. While this is an interesting observation, no other reported study has shown decline in survival for the neoadjuvant treatment approach. In addition, each of the randomized clinical studies presented above has shown no difference in local recurrence rates based upon the timing of chemotherapy adding support for the safety of neoadjuvant chemotherapy.

Another area of potential concern is determining the role of radiation therapy for patients with clinical stage I-II breast cancer who receive neoadjuvant chemotherapy. While pCR predicts improved survival, less is known about the history of patients who have residual disease after treatment. There is evidence that residual disease in the breast after neoadjuvant chemotherapy predicts a worsened prognosis compared to patients who obtain a pCR. There is also evidence that patients who achieve a pCR in the breast but have residual disease in the axilla have a worse prognosis compared to those patients who experience a pCR in both the breast and axilla [35]. The presence of residual disease also may predict in some patients for a higher risk of local recurrence- thereby lowering the threshold to administer chest wall/lymphatic radiation. Authors from M D Anderson Cancer Center evaluated patients with clinical stage I-IIIA breast cancer treated with neoadjuvant chemotherapy to assess for risk of local recurrence. They found that patients who had residual disease in the breast greater than 2.1 cm in size in conjunction with 1–3 positive lymph nodes were more likely to develop a local recurrence (30%) than patients with similar size tumor/number of involved lymph nodes who were treated with adjuvant therapy [36]. Based upon their findings, these authors conclude that radiation should be offered to patients with 4 or more lymph nodes involved with tumor, tumor size greater than 5 cm or clinical stage IIIA-IIIB breast cancer regardless of the timing of chemotherapy and the extent of tumor reduction that may occur with neoadjuvant chemotherapy. For patients with clinical stage I-II breast cancer who have T2N1 disease after neoadjuvant chemotherapy, the role of radiation therapy is controversial and should be the topic of continuing investigation.

Future Directions

Neoadjuvant chemotherapy for breast cancer used to be reserved for patients who had inoperable disease. Recent studies, however, have shown this treatment approach to be safe for patients with early-stage breast cancer and demonstrate that this treatment approach is a valuable tool for identifying effective therapies early in their development. While adjuvant chemotherapy remains the standard of care for operable breast cancer, neoadjuvant chemotherapy can help to improve the rate of breast conservation therapy by approximately 5–10%. Administration of chemotherapy prior to surgery can also potentially be used as a tool to help refine therapy for an individual. When chemotherapy is given in the adjuvant setting, it is given blindly without any ability to predict who will respond and who will ultimately have a relapse. Neoadjuvant chemotherapy allows the clinician to modify a treatment plan to avoid ineffective therapy and potentially improve upon outcome.

Recent research has focused on novel ways to identify tumor characteristics that will predict response to neoadjuvant chemotherapy. The role of estrogen receptor (ER) and progesterone receptor (PR) expression as predictors of response to neoadjuvant chemotherapy is controversial. Several studies showed a direct correlation between ER negativity and improved response [37,38], while others showed no significant correlation [39,40]. Several studies have shown a potential association between HER-2 protein overexpression and improved disease-free survival with doxorubicin-based adjuvant chemotherapy [41–43]. However, most studies have shown a limited role of HER-2 as a predictor of response to CMF [39], FAC [44,45], or taxane [40] chemotherapy in the neoadjuvant setting. Conflicting results have also been reported for the predictive role of proliferation marker Ki67 [38,40]. Other molecules under investigation include p53 [44,46], bcl-2 [47,48] and MDR-1, among others. Unfortunately, none of these markers can predict with adequate power who are the patients most likely to achieve a pCR. Gene profiling and microarray RNA analysis attempt to correlate the expression of thousands of genes found in individual breast cancers in regards with pathologic response to treatment. For example, Buchholz et al. have found that patterns of gene expression can correlate with tumor response [49]. Pusztai et al. showed that gene profiles can be generated from a single-passage fine needle aspiration [50]. Using this approach clusters of genes have been identified that strongly correlate with pCR in patients undergoing neoadjuvant therapy [51]. Future potential use would be to use these arrays to tailor a chemotherapy regimen based upon predicted response rather than the routine use of commonly applied standards.

Other potential areas of impact would be to develop minimally invasive local therapy for early-stage breast cancer to enhance breast conservation for increasing numbers of women. The use of neoadjuvant chemotherapy has expanded well beyond its initial role of necessity- making inoperable breast cancer operable. The practical and theoretical advantages associated with this treatment approach will continue to redefine our treatment for patients with operable breast cancer into the future.

REFERENCES

[1]   R. Peto, J. Boreham, M. Clarke, C. Davies and V. Beral, UK and USA breast cancer deaths down 25% in year 2000 at ages 20–69 years, *Lancet* **355**(9217) (2000), 1822.

[2]   Early Breast Cancer Trialists' Collaborative Group, Poly-chemotherapy for early breast cancer: an overview of the randomized trials, *Lancet* **352** (1998), 930–942.

[3]   Early Breast Cancer Trialists' Collaborative Group, Tamoxifen for early breast cancer. An overview of the randomized trials, *Lancet* **351** (1998), 1451–1467.

[4]   P.P. Rosen, S. Groshen and D.W. Kinne, Survival and prognostic factors in node-negative breast cancer: results of long-term follow-up studies, *J Natl Cancer Inst Monogr* (11) (1992), 159–162.

[5]   A.U. Buzdar, S.E. Singletary and V. Valero et al., Evaluation of paclitaxel in adjuvant chemotherapy for patients with operable breast cancer: preliminary data of a prospective randomized trial, *Clin Ca Res* **8** (2002), 1073–1079.

[6]   I.C. Henderson, D. Berry, G. Demetri, T. Kute, E.T. Liu, F. Koerner, C.T. Cirrincione, D.R. Budman, W.C. Wood and M. Barcos, Improved disease free (DFS) and overall survival (OS) from the addition of sequential paclitaxel (T) but not from the escalation of doxorubicin (A) dose level in the adjuvant chemotherapy of patients (PTS) with node-positive primary breast cancer (BC), *Proc Am Soc Clin Oncol* **17**(101A) (1998), Abstract 390.

[7]   J.M. Nabholtz, T. Pienkowski and J. Mackey et al., Phase III trial comparing TAC (docetaxel, doxorubicin, cyclophosphamide) with FAC (5-fluorouracil, doxorubicin, cyclophosphamide) in the adjuvant treatment of node positive breast cancer patients: interim analysis of the BCIRG 001 study, *Proc Am Soc Clin Oncol Abstract* **141** (2002).

[8]   N. Gunduz, B. Fisher and E.A. Saffer, Effect of surgical removal on the growth and kinetics of residual tumor, *Cancer Res* **39**(10) (1979), 3861–3865.

[9]   B. Fisher, N. Gunduz and E.A. Saffer, Influence of the interval between primary tumor removal and chemotherapy on kinetics and growth of metastases, *Cancer Res* **43**(4) (1983), 1488–1492.

[10]   G.N. Hortobagyi, G.R. Blumenschein and W. Spanos et al., Multimodal treatment of locoregionally advanced breast cancer, *Cancer* **51** (1983), 763–768.

[11]   G.N. Hortobagyi, S.E. Singletary and E.A. Strom, Treatment of locally advanced and inflammatory breast cancer, in: *Diseases of the Breast*, J.R. Harris, M.E. Lippman, M. Morrow and C.K. Osborne, eds, Philadelphia, Lippincott Williams and Wilkins, 2000, pp. 645–660.

[12]   C. Botti, P. Vici and M. Lopez et al., Prognostic value of lymph node metastases after neoadjuvant chemotherapy for large-size operable carcinoma of the breast, *J. Am. Coll. Surg.* **181** (1995), 202–208.

[13]   S.M. Scholl, A. Fourquet and B. Asselain et al., Neoadjuvant versus adjuvant chemotherapy in premenopausal patients with tumors considered too large for breast conserving surgery: preliminary results of a randomised trial: S6, *Eur J Cancer* **30A**(5) (1994), 645–652.

[14]   P. Broet, S.M. Sholl and A. de la Rochefordiere et al., Short and long-term effects on survival in breast cancer patients treated by primary chemotherapy: an updated analysis of a randomized trial, *Breast Cancer Res Treat* **58**(2) (1999), 151–156.

[15]   V.F. Semiglazov, E.E. Topuzov and J.L. Bavli et al., Primary (neoadjuvant) chemotherapy and radiotherapy compared with primary radiotherapy alone in stage IIb-IIIa breast cancer, *Ann Oncol* **5** (1994), 591–595.

[16]   L. Mauriac, G. MacGrogan and A. Avril et al., Neoadjuvant chemotherapy for operable breast carcinoma larger than 3 cm: a unicentre randomized trial with a 124-month median follow-up. Institut Bergonie Bordeaux Groupe Sein (IBBGS), *Ann Oncol* **10**(1) (1999), 47–52.

[17]   J. Ragaz, R. Baird and P. Rebbeck et al., Preoperative (neoadjuvant-PRE) versus postoperative (POST) adjuvant chemotherapy (CT) for stage I-II breast cancer (SI-IIBC). Long-term analysis of British Columbia randomized trial, *Proc Am Soc Clin Oncol* **16**(142a) 1997, Abstract 499.

[18]   R. Jakesz, Comparison of pre-vs. postoperative chemotherapy in breast cancer patients: four-year results of Austrian Breast and Colorectal Cancer Study Group (ABCSG) trial 7, *Proc Am Soc Clin Oncol* **20:32a** (2001), Abstract 125.

[19]   A. Makris, T.J. Powles and S.E. Ashley et al., A reduction in the requirements for mastectomy in a randomized trial of neoadjuvant chemoendocrine therapy in primary breast cancer, *Ann Oncol* **9**(11) (1998), 1179–1184.

[20]   J.A. van der Hage, C.J.H. van de Velde and J.P. Julien et al., Preoperative chemotherapy in primary operable breast cancer: results from the European organization for research and treatment of cancer trial 10902, *J Clin Oncol* **19**(22) (2001), 4224–4237.

[21]   B. Fisher, A. Brown and E. Mamounas et al., Effect of preoperative chemotherapy on local-regional disease in women with operable breast cancer: findings from national surgical adjuvant breast and bowel project B-18, *J Clin Oncol* **15**(7) (1997), 2479–2482.

[22]   B. Fisher, J. Bryant and N. Wolmark et al., Effect of preoperative chemotherapy on the outcome of women with operable breast cancer, *J Clin Oncol* **16**(8) (1998), 2672–2685.

[23]   G.N. Hortobagyi, F.C. Ames and A.U. Buzdar et al., Management of stage III primary breast cancer with primary chemotherapy, surgery and radiation therapy, *Cancer* **62**(12) (1988).

[24]   G. Bonadonna, P. Valagussa and C. Brambilla et al., Response to primary chemotherapy increases rates of breast preservation and correlates with prognosis, *Proc Am Soc Clin Oncol* **13** (1994), 107.

[25]   J.A. Sparano, Taxanes for breast cancer: an evidence-based review of randomized phase II and phase III trials, *Clin Breast Cancer* **1**(1) (2000), 32–40.

[26]   A.U. Buzdar, S.E. Singletary and R.L. Theriault et al., Prospective evaluation of paclitaxel versus combination chemotherapy with fluorouracil, doxorubicin, and cyclophosphamide as neoadjuvant therapy in patients with operable breast cancer, *J Clin Oncol* **17**(11) (1999), 3412–3417.

[27]   A.U. Buzdar, S.E. Singletary and V. Valero et al., Evaluation of paclitaxel in adjuvant chemotherapy for patients with operable breast cancer: preliminary data of a prospective randomized trial, *Clin Ca Res* **8** (2002), 1073–1079.

[28]   M.C. Green, A.U. Buzdar and T. Smith et al., Weekly paclitaxel followed by FAC as primary systemic chemotherapy of operable breast cancer improves pathologic complete remission rates when compared to every 3-week paclitaxel therapy followed by FAC- final results of a prospective phase III randomized trial, *Proc Am Soc Clin Oncol Abstract* **135** (2002).

[29]   NSABP, The effect on primary tumor response of adding sequential Taxotere to Adriamycin and cyclophosphamide: preliminary results from NSABP protocol B-27, *Breast Ca Res Treat* **69**(3) (2001), 210.

[30] I.C. Smith, H.D. Hayes and A.W. Hutcheon et al., Neoadjuvant chemotherapy in breast cancer: significantly enhanced response with docetaxel, *J Clin Oncol* **20**(6) (2002), 1456–1466.

[31] E. Thomas, A. Buzdar and G. Hortobagyi et al., Long-term follow-up of stage III breast cancer – combined modality treatment with anthracycline containing chemotherapy (CT): the M. D. Anderson experience, *Proc Am Soc Clin Oncol* **18:75a** (1999), Abstract 284.

[32] D.A. Mankoff, L.K. Dunnwald and J.R. Gralow et al., Blood flow and metabolism in locally advanced breast cancer: relationship with response to therapy, *J Nucl Med* **43**(4) (2002), 500–509.

[33] K. Wasser, K. Klein and C. Fink et al., Evaluation of neoadjuvant chemotherapeutic response of breast cancer using dynamic MRI with high temporal resolution, *Eur Radiol* **13**(1) (2003), 80–87.

[34] S.C. Partridge, J.E. Gibbs and Y. Lu et al., Accuracy of MR imaging for revealing residual breast cancer in patients who have undergone neoadjuvant chemotherapy, *Am J Roentgenol* **179**(5) (2002), 1193–1199.

[35] M.R. Machiavelli, A.O. Romero and J.E. Perez et al., Prognostic significance of pathological response of primary tumor and metastatic axillary lymph nodes after neoadjuvant chemotherapy for locally advanced breast cancer, *Cancer J Sci Am* **4**(2) (1998), 125–131.

[36] T.A. Buchholz, A. Katz and E.A. Strom et al., Pathologic tumor size and lymph node status predict for different rates of localregional recurrence after mastectomy for breast cancer patients treated with neoadjuvant versus adjuvant therapy, *Int J Radiat Oncol Biol Phys* **53**(4) (2002), 880–888.

[37] J. Chang, T.J. Powles, D.C. Allred, S.E. Ashley, G.M. Clark and A. Makris et al., Biologic markers as predictors of clinical outcome from systemic therapy for primary operable breast cancer, *J Clin Oncol* **17** (1999), 3058–3063.

[38] G. MacGrogan, L. Mauriac, M. Durand, F. Bonichon, M. Trojani, M.I. de and J.M. Coindre, Primary chemotherapy in breast invasive carcinoma: predictive value of the immunohistochemical detection of hormonal receptors, p53, c-erbB-2, MiB1, pS2 and GST pi, *Brit J Cancer* **74** (1996), 1458–1465.

[39] A. Bottini, A. Berruti, A. Bersiga, A. Brunelli, M.P. Brizzi and B.D. Marco et al., Effect of neoadjuvant chemotherapy on Ki67 labelling index, c-erbB-2 expression and steroid hormone receptor status in human breast tumours, *Anticancer Res* **16** (1996), 3105–3110.

[40] L.G. Estevez, J.M. Cuevas, A. Anton, J. Florian, J.M. Lopez-Vega, A. Velasco, F. Lobo, A. Herrero and J. Fortes, Weekly docetaxel as neoadjuvant chemotherapy for stage II and III breast cancer: efficacy and correlation with biological markers in a phase II, multicenter study, *Clin Cancer Res* **9**(2) (2003), 686–692.

[41] S. Paik, J. Bryant and C. Park et al., erbB-2 and response to doxorubicin in patients with axillary lymph node-positive, hormone receptor-negative breast cancer, *J Natl Cancer Inst* **90** (1998), 1361–1370.

[42] A.D. Thor, D.A. Berry and D.R. Budman et al., erbB-2, p53, and efficacy of adjuvant therapy in lymph node-positive breast cancer, *J Natl Cancer Inst* **90** (1998), 1346–1360.

[43] A. Moliterni, S. Menard, P. Valagussa, E. Biganzoli, P. Boracchi, A. Balsari, P. Casalini, G. Tomasic, E. Marubini, S. Pilotti and G. Bonadonna, HER2 Overexpression and Doxorubicin in Adjuvant Chemotherapy for Resectable Breast Cancer, *J Clin Oncol* **21**(3) (2003), 458–462.

[44] S. Rozan, A. Vincent-Salomon, B. Zafrani, P. Validire, P. De Cremoux and Bernoux et al., No significant predictive value of c-erbB-2 or p53 expression regarding sensitivity to primary chemotherapy or radiotherapy in breast cancer, *Int J Cancer* **79** (1998), 27–33.

[45] F. Zhang, L. Pusztai, Y. Yang, T. Smith, S-W. Kau, J. McConathy, F.J. Esteva and G.N. Hortobagyi, Correlation between HER2 expression of breast cancer and response to neoadjuvant FAC chemotherapy, *Proc Am Soc Clin Oncol* **21:32a** (2002), Abstract 124.

[46] S.C. Formenti, G. Dunnington, B. Uzieli, H. Lenz, S. Keren-Rosenberg and H. Silberman et al., Original p53 status predicts for pathological response in locally advanced breast cancer patients treated preoperatively with continuous infusion 5-fluorouracil and radiation therapy, *Int J Radiat Oncol Biol Phys* **39** (1997), 1059–1068.

[47] L. Pusztai, S. Krishnamurthy, J. Perez-Cardona, N. Sneige, F.J. Esteva, M. Volchenok, P. Breitenfelder, S.W. Kau, S. Takayama, S. Krajewski, J.C. Reed, G.N. Hortobagyi and R.C. Bast, Expression of BAG-1 and BCL-2 proteins before and after neoadjuvant chemotherapy of locally advanced breast cancer, *Cancer Investigation*, in press.

[48] T.A. Buchholz, D. Davis, D.J. McConkey, W.F. Symmans, V. Valero, A. Jhingran, S.L. Tucker, L. Pusztai, M. Cristofanilli, F.J. Esteva, G.N. Hortobagyi and A.A. Sahin, Chemotherapy-induced apoptosis and bcl-2 levels correlated with breast cancer response, *Cancer J*, in press.

[49] T. Buchholz, D.N. Stivers and J. Stec et al., Global gene expression changes during neoadjuvant chemotherapy for human breast cancer, *Cancer J* **8** (2002), 461–468.

[50] Pusztai, M. Ayers, J. Stec, E. Clark, K. Hess, D. Stivers, A. Damokosh, N. Sneige, T.A. Buchholz, F.J. Esteva, B. Arun, D. Booser, M. Rosales, V. Valero, C. Adams, G.N. Hortobagyi and W.F. Symmans, Gene expression profiles obtained from single passage fine needle aspirations (FNA) of breast cancer reliably identify prognostic/predictive markers such as estrogen (ER) and HER-2 receptor status and reveal large scale molecular differences between ER-negative and ER-positive tumors, *Clin Cancer Res*, in press.

[51] M. Ayers, W.F. Symmans, J. Stec, J. Metivier, A. Damokosh, E. Clark, N. Sneige, C. Carter, G. Whitman, G.H. Hortobagyi and L. Pusztai, Gene expression profiling of fine needle aspirations of breast cancer identifies genes associated with complete pathologic response to neoadjuvant taxol/FAC chemotherapy, *Breast Cancer Res Treat* **76**(1):S64, (2002), Abst 220.

Breast Disease 21 (2004) 33–40
IOS Press

When Not to Treat – Chemotherapy for Small ($\leq$ 1 cm) Breast Cancers

Sharon E. Soule*
Indiana University School of Medicine, Indianapolis, IN, USA

Abstract. The role of adjuvant chemotherapy in treatment of breast cancers $\leq$ 1.0 cm is controversial. Careful consideration must be given to the patient's overall risk of recurrence and death given her tumor size and lymph node status. Studies indicate that overall survival for women with lymph node-negative breast cancers $\leq$ 1.0 cm is 90–99%. Given the known relative benefit of adjuvant chemotherapy for breast cancer, the absolute benefit of chemotherapy in this setting is usually $\leq$ 1%. The toxicities of adjuvant chemotherapy, including cognitive dysfunction, early menopause, cardiac dysfunction, and leukemia, are significant to patients. The decision to treat women who are already at a very low risk of recurrence with adjuvant chemotherapy must involve an honest and detailed discussion between the patient and her oncologist.

INTRODUCTION

The use of adjuvant chemotherapy to eliminate microscopic metastases and thereby decrease the risk of breast cancer recurrence and death was first studied in the late 1960s and early 1970s. A National Surgical Adjuvant Breast and Bowel Project (NSABP) trial found improved disease-free survival in premenopausal women with lymph node metastases who were treated with adjuvant L-PAM therapy [1]. Shortly thereafter, a study by the Milan Istituto Nazionale per lo Studio e la Cura dei Tumori documented a survival advantage with adjuvant cyclophosphamide, methotrexate and 5-fluorouracil (CMF) in premenopausal, lymph node-positive women [2]. At that time, adjuvant chemotherapy for lymph node-negative or post-menopausal women was thought not justified due to their more favorable prognosis and the toxicities of chemotherapy. Indeed, a 1985 NIH consensus conference recommended that women without lymph node metastases should not receive adjuvant chemotherapy [3].

Might this benefit extend to women without lymph node metastases? In 1989, NSABP B-13 found improved disease-free and overall survival with the use of methotrexate and fluorouracil (MF) compared to placebo in patients with lymph node-negative tumors [4]. Accordingly, the 1990 NIH consensus conference reversed the previous recommendations regarding chemotherapy in women without lymph node metastases [5]. The survival advantage was later confirmed by NSABP B-19, which randomized women without lymph node metastases to CMF versus sequential MF. Patients treated with CMF experienced an increase in overall survival and disease-free survival [6].

In the past three decades, literally hundreds of randomized controlled trials have been performed examining the role of adjuvant chemotherapy. The sheer number of trials and at times contradictory results lead the Early Breast Cancer Trialists' Collaborative Group (EBCTCG) to perform a regular meta-analysis of available randomized controlled trials. This meta-analysis offers the practicing physician a sense of the broad trends in adjuvant therapy. In the most recent EBCTCG analysis, combination chemotherapy produced a 23.5% relative reduction in the annual hazard of recurrence ($2p < 0.00001$), and a 15.3% relative reduction in the annual hazard of death ($2p < 0.00001$) [7].

Though the *relative* benefits of adjuvant therapy are independent of nodal status, the *absolute* reduction in

---

*Address for correspondence: Dr. Soule, 535 Barnhill Drive, RT-473, Indianapolis, Indiana 46202, USA. Tel.: +1 317 278 6942; Fax: +1 317 274 3646; E-mail: shsoule@iupui.edu.

relapse and death will be greatest in high-risk patients and smallest in low-risk patients. For instance, a 20% relative risk reduction for a patient with a baseline 50% risk of recurrence will result in an absolute reduction of 10% (i.e., from 50% to 40%). Alternatively a patient with a 10% baseline risk of recurrence will reduce her risk of recurrence to 8%, a 2% absolute reduction. As no breast cancer patient has a zero risk of recurrence or death, each will derive some (perhaps miniscule) benefit from adjuvant therapy.

Which patients have such a small absolute benefit from adjuvant therapy that this benefit is outweighed by the treatment toxicity? The increasing use of mammography and the subsequent increase in detection of tumors $\leqslant 1$ cm in greatest diameter $(T_{1a-b}N_0M_0)$ has led clinicians to face this issue more frequently. To address this controversial topic, the article will first present data regarding the prognosis of patients with tumors $\leqslant 1$ cm. Further discussion will involve the known risk of adjuvant therapy to the patient, followed by analysis of issues pertaining to age and comorbidity. Also pertinent to this discussion is a consideration of the biases of both patients and physicians when discussing and making decisions about adjuvant therapy in this setting.

PROGNOSIS FOR WOMEN WITH SMALL TUMORS

Relative reductions in the rate of recurrence and mortality must be considered within the overall context of a patient's baseline risk of recurrence or death due to her particular cancer. A relative survival benefit may become minimally significant if the overall risk of death due to breast cancer is extremely low. Therefore, it is important to define the risk of recurrence and death due to small tumors in order to apply the benefit of adjuvant therapy to that specific situation. Multiple studies have attempted to define the risk of recurrence and death for women with breast cancers $\leqslant 1.0$ cm (Table 1).

The Surveillance, Epidemiology, and End Results (SEER) Program of the National Cancer Institute has collected data on cancer survival for nearly 10% of the United States population since 1973. Tumor size and axillary lymph node involvement were assessed in 24,740 women with breast cancer between 1977 and 1982. Tumors <1.0 cm in diameter comprised 5.4% of all tumors; of these, 79.4% were lymph node negative $(T_{1a,b}N_0M_0)$. All patients with lymph-node negative tumors smaller than 2 cm had a 5-year survival rate of

96.3%. Five-year survival was 98.3% for women with tumors 0.5–0.9 cm in diameter. Patients with tumors < 0.5 cm had an average survival of 99.2% [8].

Rosen et al., evaluated 767 women with early stage breast cancer treated from 1964 through 1970 with surgical therapy alone. After more than 20 years of follow-up, 10 year recurrence-free survival (RFS) for the 171 patients with tumors $\leqslant 1.0$ cm was 91%; RFS at 20 years was 88%. Recurrence-free survival was influenced significantly by both the size of the primary tumor and the histologic classification. $T_1N_0M_0$ tumors with favorable histologic subtypes, including medullary, mucinous, papillary, tubular and adenocystic, had a 5% recurrence rate, with no deaths due to breast cancer. In the group of patients with tumors $\leqslant 1.0$ cm, the probability of dying of cardiovascular disease or second non-breast malignancies was equal to the risk of death due to ipsilateral breast carcinoma [9].

Leitner et al., retrospectively reviewed 218 patients with lymph node-negative breast cancer $\leqslant 1.0$ cm to determine prognosis and to identify useful prognostic factors. Only nine of these patients had been treated with adjuvant chemotherapy. Thirty-one percent had tumors $\leqslant 0.5$ cm (T_{1a}); the remaining 69% were > 0.5 cm but $\leqslant 1.0$ cm (T_{1b}). Relapse-free survival at seven years for T_{1a} tumors was 98%; relapse-free survival for T_{1b} tumors was 90%. Recurrence-free survival for all patients at 7 years was 93%. Prognostic factors associated with a higher risk of relapse included tumor size, poor histologic grade, poor nuclear grade and lymphatic vessel invasion. The combination of poor nuclear grade and lymphatic vessel invasion were the most predictive of a poor outcome in a multivariate analysis. This combination of factors was found in 10% of patients and resulted in a 67% recurrence-free survival [10].

Another study pertinent to this topic is a retrospective analysis of 1329 women diagnosed with lymph node-negative breast cancer between 1991 and 1992. It was found that, of 70% of those patients with Stage I disease, 37% had tumors $\leqslant 1.0$ cm; 5-year disease-free survival in this subset of patients was 94%. For a further subgroup of these women with tumors $\leqslant 1.0$ cm that were also estrogen receptor positive and histologic Grade I, the 5-year disease-free survival was 97% [11].

The Danish Breast Cancer Group registry, inclusive of virtually all Danes with breast cancer, performed a retrospective analysis of 30,000 women with breast cancer, in an attempt to identify a group with sufficiently low risk as to avoid chemotherapy. Premenopausal women with receptor-positive, node-

Table 1
Prognosis of patients with tumors $\leqslant 1$ cm

Study	Pts.	F/U (yrs.)	RFS (%)			OS (%)			Systemic Rx.
Tumor size (cm)			< 0.5	0.5–0.9	$\leqslant 1.0$	< 0.5	0.5–0.9	$\leqslant 1.0$	
SEER	1060	5				99.2	98.3	96.3*	unknown
Rosen	171	10			91				none
		20			88				
Leitner	218	6.9	98	90	93				chemotherapy – 9 pts.
Proc ASCO	344	9–10			94				unknown
Danish, ER+, Grade I	6000	5						98*	none
BCDDP (Seidman)	880	8						95	unknown
Swedish (Arnesson)	254	7						98.7	tamoxifen – 8%
Lee	87	7.8	100		92	100		98	Hormonal tx – 17%
NSABP, ER-	61	8			81			93	none
	174				90			91	chemotherapy
NSABP, ER+	264	8			86			90	none
	540				93			92	tamoxifen
	220				95			97	tam + chemo

*All tumors < 2.0 cm.

negative grade I (Bloom-Richardson grading) cancers treated with local therapy only had a 5-year survival rate of 98%, identical to that of age-matched controls. Similarly, in postmenopausal women 5-year survival was 91% for the breast cancer cohort and 92% for age-matched controls [12].

Three smaller studies of patients with tumors $\leqslant$ 1.0 cm include the Breast Cancer Detection Demonstration Project (BCDDP), a series from the Swedish Mammography Screening Program, and a series by Lee, et al., The BCDDP reported a 95% 5-year survival for stage I cancers $\leqslant$ 1.0 cm. Although it was likely to be low, the actual number of patients in this series who received systemic therapy is unknown [13]. Three hundred twenty-four women in the Swedish study with breast cancers $\leqslant$ 1.0 cm in diameter were treated with surgery and/or radiotherapy. None of the patients received cytotoxic therapy; 8% of patients were treated with tamoxifen. Lymph node metastases were present in 12% of patients. Recurrence-free survival in patients without lymph node metastases was 99%; overall recurrence-free survival was 97% [14]. Lee, et al studied 87 women with lymph node-negative breast cancers that were $\leqslant$ 1.0 cm [15]. Disease-free survival rate was 92%; overall survival was 98%, although two patients were alive but with bone metastases at the time of analysis.

Finally, retrospective subset analysis of 1259 patients with tumors $\leqslant$ 1.0 cm enrolled in multiple adjuvant trials conducted by the NSABP has suggested that a small but real fraction of such patients will reduce their risk of recurrence through the use of adjuvant chemotherapy. The 8-year recurrence-free survival for women with ER-negative tumors of < 1 cm treated with surgery alone or with surgery plus chemotherapy were 81% and 90%, respectively ($p = 0.06$), though survival was identical (93 and 91%). Among women with ER-positive tumors < 1 cm receiving tamoxifen, a similar pattern was seen, with 8-year relapse-free survival rates of 86% (surgery alone), 93% (surgery plus Tamoxifen) and 95% (surgery plus Tamoxifen plus chemotherapy). Survival rates for the three groups were 90%, 92%, and 97%, respectively ($p = 0.01$). The authors' conclusion as a result of this study was that the use of chemotherapy and/or tamoxifen should be considered for women with tumors $\leqslant$ 1.0 cm and no axillary lymph node metastases [16].

It is difficult to reconcile the results of the NSABP with population-based or registry results from other groups. First, 60% of tumors in the NSABP series were exactly 1.0 cm in diameter, bringing the accuracy of tumor measurements into question. This suggests a "grouping effect" with rounding of tumor size rather than exact measurements. Event-free survival data in the NSABP study included ipsilateral recurrences and new contralateral breast cancers as events; these were not usually included in the other series. Despite the differences in tumor measurement and reporting procedures, the role of selection bias can not be ignored. Physicians enroll particular "low-risk" patients on adjuvant chemotherapy trials because they do not perceive these patients as being at low risk. Some combination of pathologic factors often influences the physician's gestalt in ways that are not easily measurable.

RISKS OF ADJUVANT THERAPY

A risk-benefit analysis of adjuvant therapy must include consideration of both acute and chronic toxicities of chemotherapy and endocrine therapy. Death due to adjuvant chemotherapy is rare, but when it occurs, it is usually due to thromboembolic events or neutropenic sepsis. There were no toxicity-related deaths among the approximately 2,000 patients treated with doxorubicin and cyclophosphamide (AC) or CMF adjuvant therapy in the NSABP B-15 trial [17]. Nine treatment-related deaths occurred among 966 patients treated with CMF and tamoxifen in an Intergroup trial [18]. Overall lethal toxicities occur in approximately one of every 200 to 500 women who are treated with adjuvant chemotherapy [19]. Deaths are more common in post-menopausal patients and in patients receiving concurrent tamoxifen therapy. Less severe but more common acute toxicities of adjuvant chemotherapy for breast cancer include alopecia, nausea and vomiting, anemia, thrombocytopenia and fatigue.

CARDIAC DYSFUNCTION

Although adjuvant chemotherapy is generally well tolerated, there are some serious long-term toxicities. Cardiomyopathy is a known toxicity of anthracycline-based chemotherapy. Cardiac dysfunction correlates with the cumulative dose of doxorubicin and patient age; it is rare when the dose is limited to $< 300\ \mathrm{mg/m}^2$ in patients under the age of 65. A recent cohort study of women with Stage I and II breast cancer demonstrates that the incidence of heart disease increases from a relatively infrequent 7.1% incidence in women aged 65–74 to the quite common 21.2% incidence in women aged 75–84. Long-term cardiac effects occurring 11 years after adjuvant doxorubicin therapy, measured by systolic dysfunction, were identified in 7.9% of patients [20]. The incidence of cardiac dysfunction may be further limited by the use of continuous infusion of doxorubicin, though at the expense of added inconvenience and cost [21].

MYELODYSPLASTIC SYNDROME/LEUKEMIA

Treatment-related myelodysplastic syndrome (MDS) and leukemia are rare but devastating long-term side effects of chemotherapy. A study analyzed the incidence of leukemias in 1,474 women enrolled in clinical trials and treated with FAC-based chemotherapy at M.D. Anderson Cancer Center between 1974 and 1989. At 10 years of follow-up, 14 patients (1.5%) were identified who subsequently developed acute myelogenous leukemia (5 patients), MDS (8 patients) and chronic myelogenous leukemia (1 patient). Six of these patients had chromosomal abnormalities characteristic of leukemias resulting from treatment with alkylating agents. Twelve patients had received both chemotherapy and radiation therapy; two received chemotherapy alone [22]. Escalating the dose of cyclophosphamide clearly increases this risk of treatment-related leukemia. Sixteen patients (0.87%) enrolled on NSABP B-25 have been diagnosed with myelodysplastic syndrome or acute myelogenous leukemia. Nine of these patients had cytogenetic abnormalities associated with secondary leukemias [23].

The incidence of acute leukemia or myelodysplastic syndrome diagnosed in patients treated on six trials of adjuvant chemotherapy conducted by the Eastern Cooperative Oncology Group between 1978 and 1987 has also been reported. Included were 2,638 patients treated with cyclophosphamide-based chemotherapy; only 130 patients received adjuvant radiotherapy. Three patients were subsequently diagnosed with MDS, one developed AML and another developed a T-cell ALL. The overall incidence of hematologic malignancies in this group was 0.2%, which was similar to that observed in the general population. However, confidence intervals for these numbers are wide; therefore definite conclusions are difficult [24]. In these studies of treatment-related hematologic disorders, the incidence is also statistically higher in patients who receive chemotherapy and radiotherapy versus patients treated with chemotherapy alone. This could explain the lower incidence of hematologic malignancies in the ECOG study.

PREMATURE OVARIAN FAILURE

Premature ovarian failure is another important effect of adjuvant chemotherapy. Thirty-five percent of women under 40 years old who receive 6 cycles of CMF will suffer premature menopause compared with 90% of women over the age of 40. The incidence after four cycles of AC is 13% in women under 40 and 60% in women over 40 years old [25]. A study of 35 women who underwent early menopause after adjuvant chemotherapy for breast cancer evaluated bone loss at 6 and 12 months after starting chemotherapy. There was a statistically significant decline of 3.7% in bone mineral density at the 12-month evaluation for this group of women. The 14 women who retained ovarian function had no decrease in bone mineral density [26]. Although this study did not address clinical endpoints, it is likely that this translates into a significant risk of osteoporosis due to premature ovarian failure. A similar study shows average bone mineral density values in women who became amenorrheic due to chemotherapy to be 10% lower than that in age-matched controls [27]. Bothersome menopausal symptoms such as hot flashes, vaginal dryness and mood swings, while not life-threatening, certainly also have a negative impact on quality of life.

COGNITIVE DYSFUNCTION

Another emerging concern is the increasing evidence for cognitive deficits in patients receiving chemotherapy, especially in women treated for breast cancer. Although patients have complained for years about changes in cognitive function during adjuvant therapy, only recently has this area been subjected to careful, randomized study. How common is 'chemo brain'? Are the effects transient or permanent?

Investigators at the Princess Margaret Hospital reported results of a matched cohort study comparing women receiving chemotherapy for breast cancer and women without cancer [28,29]. Women < 60 years old who had received at least three cycles of adjuvant chemotherapy recruited a friend of similar age for the control group. All subjects completed High-Sensitivity Cognitive Screen and FACT-G QL scale with sub-scales for endocrine function and fatigue. Data is now available for the initial evaluation in 186 of 200 women; further assessments are planned for the entire group at one and two years later. Patients experienced significantly more fatigue (FACT-F scores of 46 vs. 31, $p < 0.0001$), menopausal symptoms (FACT-ES scores of 64 vs 58, $p < 0.0001$) and global quality of life symptoms (FACT-G scores of 93 vs 76, $p < 0.0001$) compared with control women. In addition, the incidence of moderate to severe cognitive dysfunction was 16% in patients versus 4% in the control population ($p = 0.001$), independent of fatigue and menopausal symptoms.

Another study performed at Princess Margaret Hospital involved 107 women: 31 currently receiving adjuvant chemotherapy (CEF or CMF), 40 who completed adjuvant chemotherapy at least one year prior to enrollment, and 36 healthy female controls [30]. These women were assessed using the High Sensitivity Cognitive Screen (HSCS), testing memory, language, visual-motor, spatial, attention and concentration, and self-regulation and planning. The median total HSCS scores were statistically different between the women currently receiving chemotherapy and the healthy controls (37.0 versus 26.0, $p = 0.009$). More women in

both treatment groups had significantly increased moderate or severe cognitive impairment compared with the control women. There were no significant differences among the three groups for mood disturbance parameters.

In addition to the above studies of the short-term impact of chemotherapy, a study by Ahles, et al, involved long-term cognitive evaluation of survivors of breast cancer and lymphoma [31]. Seventy-one patients (35 breast cancer, 36 lymphoma) who received systemic chemotherapy and 57 patients (35 breast cancer, 22 lymphoma) treated with local therapy alone who were disease-free for a minimum of 5 years after diagnosis were included. These patients were then assessed using a battery of standardized neuropsychological tests. Using multivariate analysis, patients who received systemic chemotherapy scored significantly lower than those who did not receive systemic therapy ($p < 0.04$) overall; univariate analysis revealed significant differences in verbal memory ($p < 0.01$) and psychomotor functioning ($P < 0.03$).

Therefore, there is increasing data that chemotherapy-induced cognitive dysfunction is a reality, but how long does it actually last? The Ahles data suggest that these changes may persist for years. Follow-up of an earlier study of cognitive dysfunction has also attempted to answer this question. Schagen, et al. initially had compared thirty-nine patients with axillary lymph node-positive breast cancer treated with adjuvant CMF and tamoxifen with 34 age-matched patients who received no adjuvant chemotherapy. Patients were evaluated with 14 neuropsychologic tests as well as quality of life assessment using the EORTC QLQ-C30 questionnaire. The incidence of cognitive impairment for patients treated with chemotherapy was 28% compared with 12% in the control group. Patients treated with chemotherapy also reported more problems with concentration (31% versus 6%) and with memory (21% versus 3%) [32]. In a separate study, they also evaluated 23 patients who had received FEC chemotherapy and 22 patients who had received five cycles of FEC chemotherapy $\pm$ autologous stem cell transplant, all of whom had undergone similar cognitive analyses as part of another clinical trial [33]. Patients from both studies who had not experienced relapse of breast cancer or other new neurological or psychiatric conditions were then re-evaluated at 4 years post-therapy. Although the results may be skewed by attrition rates and small sample sizes, it was encouraging that patients in all chemotherapy groups were found to have improvement in all measurements of cognitive dysfunction [34]. Although these results are promising, they will need to be confirmed by larger prospectively designed studies.

AGE AND COMORBIDITY

is seen with each advancing decade. Although the reason for this decrement is unclear, it is certain that age and morbidity often coexist. Comorbidity represents (and properly so) a significant hurdle to achieving therapeutic efficacy. Yancik and colleagues examined a cohort of postmenopausal breast cancer patients aged 55 and older to measure their incidence of comorbid conditions. Because these women were randomly selected from several tumor registries, they were a more representative sample than the highly select patients entering clinical trials. While fewer than 20% of women in the age 55–59 group have one or more serious comorbid conditions, more than 50% of women over age 80 have one or more serious comorbidities. If one examines causes of death in this study, the percentage of women dying of breast cancer decreases steadily with advancing age: while 75% of deaths in the age 55–64 group resulted from breast cancer, only 27.6% of deaths in women aged 85 and older were breast cancer-related [35].

Comorbidity is related to age, yet also age-independent. Investigators examining the SEER database in Detroit addressed the statistical association between comorbidity and cause of death in patients with early stage breast cancer [36]. They developed a comorbidity index based on the presence of seven factors: myocardial infarction, other heart disease, diabetes, other cancers, respiratory illness, gallbladder disease, and liver conditions. As the number of conditions increased, the relative likelihood of a patient dying of breast cancer decreased. With no comorbid conditions, a patient was 4.1-fold more likely to die of breast cancer than another cause. By the time a patient had three or more comorbid conditions, the ratio of breast cancer deaths to other deaths declined to 0.3. Adjusted all-cause 3-year mortality rate was 188.4/1000 for 3+ versus 47.7/1000 person-years for zero comorbid conditions.

PHYSICIAN AND PATIENT BIASES

Assisting a patient in understanding her risk of recurrence of breast cancer is not an easy task and is one that can be easily (and perhaps dangerously) swayed by her oncologist's bias. Tannock and colleagues surveyed 307 American and European oncologists. The clinicians were asked if they would recommend adjuvant chemotherapy to women in each of two scenar-

ios involving estrogen receptor negative breast cancer. They were also asked to state the percentage of clinical benefit they required to justify the therapy. Comparison of the oncologists' response with data from the recently published EBCTCG analysis found that oncologists overestimated the improvement in relapse-free survival by twice the actual level and the improvement in overall survival by three times the reported value. This data warns that oncologists tend to be unrealistic about the benefit a breast cancer patient derives from adjuvant chemotherapy. One must assume that this misconception is commonly presented to patients as well [37].

Patients also tend to overestimate the value of adjuvant therapy. A study published in 1998 reported the results of a survey sent to breast cancer survivors; responses were received from 318 women who had received adjuvant chemotherapy. The median age of respondents was 49 years; 65% were college educated. Of the 68% of patients who reported on their understanding of risk of relapse, the median estimate of absolute benefit from adjuvant chemotherapy was 30%. These women also overestimated their risk of recurrence at 5 years by more than 100%. In addition, only 31% of women reported that they were given quantitative information about their prognosis, with or without chemotherapy [38]. Patients were also asked to quantify the minimal acceptable benefit to justify the use of adjuvant chemotherapy. Interestingly, allowable reduction in recurrence risk for respondents was 0.5% to 1%, an absolute benefit unlikely for a patient with a baseline risk of < 5%.

Discussions of adjuvant therapy in the medical literature frequently ignore patient preference. This is unfortunate, for real-world discussions of adjuvant therapy often involve complex negotiations between patient and physician. A study by Lindley, et al., of 86 patients with early-stage breast cancer found that 65% of patients will accept adjuvant chemotherapy for a 5% improvement in overall survival, suggesting that a significant minority will not. Similarly, 47% of these women were willing to receive 6 months of adjuvant chemotherapy if an additional 3 months of survival could be gained, therefore 53% were not willing to accept this treatment. Acceptance of chemotherapy for a given benefit was directly related to the disruption of women's normal lives due to chemotherapy treatments [39]. Levine, et al., reported that patient preference is dependent both on likelihood of benefit and the potential for toxicity; as benefit decreases and toxicity increases, a patient's desire to receive adjuvant chemotherapy decreases [40].

CONCLUSION

With full knowledge of the risks and benefits of chemotherapy for this subset of breast cancer patients with excellent prognosis, the answer as to whether adjuvant chemotherapy is appropriate will differ based on the age, comorbidities, pathologic characterisitcs and individual attitudes of each patient. It is the difficult role of the oncologist to present each patient with accurate data regarding her overall risk of recurrence and death from her breast cancer. A joint decision must then be reached based on the patient's realistic understanding of her situation and her wishes regarding further treatment. Novel approaches to decision making, such as the computer-assisted approach by Ravdin and colleagues, may improve physician's ability to tailor appropriate therapy to the individual patient's preference [41].

Unfortunately, because of the complexities of conflicting trial data, potential long-term toxicity, variable comorbidities and patient preferences, absolute rules for the use of adjuvant therapy for small tumors should not be universally applied. Clinical trials are relatively clean and well-defined, while actual discussions with patients are often much more complex and difficult. The art of medicine involves weighing risk and benefit, discussing pros and cons, and helping each patient to make an informed decision regarding her treatment.

REFERENCES

[1]　B. Fisher, P. Carbone, S.G. Economou et al., L-Phenylalanine mustard (L-PAM) in the management of primary breast cancer: a report of early findings, *N Engl J Med* **292** (1975), 117–122.

[2]　G. Bonadonna, P. Valagussa, A. Moliterni et al., Adjuvant cyclophosphamide, methotrexate and fluorouracil in node-positive breast cancer: the results of 20 years of follow-up, *N Engl J Med* **332** (1995), 901–906.

[3]　Adjuvant Chemotherapy for Breast Cancer, *NIH Consensus Statement Online* **5**(12) (Sep 9–11 1985), 1–19.

[4]　B. Fisher, J. Dignam, E.P. Mamounas et al., Sequential methotrexate and fluorouracil for the treatment of node-negative breast cancer patients with estrogen receptor-negative tumors: eight-year results from National Surgical Adjuvant Breast and Bowel Project (NSABP) B-13 and first report of findings from NSABP B-19 comparing methotrexate and fluorouracil with conventional cyclophosphamide, methotrexate and fluorouracil, *J Clin Oncol* **14** (1996), 1982–1992.

[5]　Treatment of Early Stage Breast Cancer, *NIH Consensus Statement Online* **8**(6) (June 18-21 1990), 1–19.

[6]　B. Fisher, J. Dignam, E.P. Mamounas et al., Sequential methotrexate and fluorouracil for the treatment of node-negative breast cancer patients with estrogen receptor-negative tumors: eight-year results from National Surgical Adjuvant Breast and Bowel Project (NSABP) B-19 comparing methotrexate and fluorouracil with conventional cyclophosphamide, methotrexate and fluorouracil, *J Clin Oncol* **14** (1996), 1982.

[7]　Early Breast Cancer Trialists' Collaborative Group: Polychemotherapy for early breast cancer: an overview of the randomized trials, *The Lancet* **352** (1998), 930–942.

[8]　C. Carter, C. Allen and D. Henson, Relation of tumor size, lymph node status, and survival in 24,740 breast cancer cases, *Cancer* **63** (1989), 181–187.

[9]　P. Rosen, S. Groshen, D. Kinne et al., Factors influencing prognosis in node-negative breast carcinoma: Analysis of 767 T1N0M0/T2N0M0 patients with long-term follow-up, *J Clin Oncol* **11** (1993), 2090–2100.

[10]　S. Leitner, A. Swern, D. Weinberger et al., Predictors of recurrence for patients with small (one centimeter or less) localized breast cancer ($T_{1a,b}N_0M_0$), *Cancer* **76** (1995), 2266–2274.

[11]　H. Joensuu, M. Lundin, K. Holli et al., Selection criteria for the low-risk subgroup in T1N0M0 breast cancer: a nationwide cohort study, *Proc. ASCO* **20** (2001), 121.

[12]　Danish Breast Cancer Group (DBCG) May 2000, Newsletter 32.

[13]　H. Seidman, S.K. Gelb, E. Silverberg et al., Survival experience in the Breast Cancer Detection Demonstration Project, *CA Cancer J Clin* **37** (1987), 258–290.

[14]　L. Arnesson, S. Smeds and G. Fagerberg, Recurrence-free survival in patients with small breast cancers, *Eur J Surg* **160** (1994), 271–276.

[15]　A.K. Lee, M. Loda, G. Mackarem et al., Lymph Node Negative Invasive Breast Carcinoma 1 Centimeter or Less in Size ($T_{1a,b}N_0M_0$), *Cancer* **79**(4) (1997), 761–771.

[16]　B. Fisher, J. Dignam, E. Tan-Chiu et al., Prognosis and treatment of patients with breast tumors of one centimeter or less and negative axillary lymph nodes, *J Natl Cancer Inst* **93** (2001), 112–120.

[17]　B. Fisher, A.M. Brown, N.V. Dimitrov et al., Two months of doxorubicin-cyclophosphamide with and without interval reinduction therapy compared with 6 months of cyclophosphamide, methotrexate, and fluorouracil in positive-node breast cancer patients with tamoxifen-nonresponsive tumors: results from the National Surgical Adjuvant Breast and Bowel Project B-15, *J Clin Oncol* **8** (1990), 1483.

[18]　H.C. Falkson, R. Gray, W.H. Wolberg et al., Adjuvant trial of 12 cycles of CMFPT followed by observation or continuous tamoxifen versus four cycles of CMFPT in postmenopausal women with breast cancer: an Eastern Cooperative Oncology Group Phase III Study, *J Clin Oncol* **8** (1990), 599.

[19]　C. Osborne and P. Ravdin, Adjuvant Systemic Therapy of Primary Breast Cancer, in: *Diseases of the Breast*, J. Harris, M. Lippman, M. Morrow and C. Osborne, eds, Philadelphia: Lippincott Williams & Wilkins; 2000, pp. 599–632.

[20]　L. Gianni, M. Zambetti, A. Moliterni et al., Cardiac sequelae in operable breast cancer patients after CMF $\pm$ doxorubicin (A) $\pm$ irradiation (abstract), *Proc ASCO* **18** (1999), 68a.

[21]　G. Hortobagyi, D. Frye, A. Buzdar et al., Decreased cardiac toxicity of doxorubicin administered by continuous intravenous infusion in combination chemotherapy for metastatic breast carcinoma, *Cancer* **63** (1989), 37–45.

[22]　E. Diamandidou, A. Buzdar, T. Smith et al., Treatment-related leukemia in breast cancer patients treated with fluorouracil-doxorubicin-cyclopho sphamide combination adjuvant chemotherapy: The University of Texas M.D. Anderson Cancer Center experience, *J Clin Oncol* **14** (1996), 2722–2730.

[23] A. DeCillis, S. Anderson, J. Bryant et al., Acute myeloid leukemia (AML) and myelodysplastic syndrome (MDS) on NSABP B-25: an update, *Proc ASCO* **16** (1997), 459.

[24] M. Tallman, R. Gray, J. Bennett et al., Leukemogenic potential of adjuvant chemotherapy for early-stage breast cancer: The Eastern Cooperative Oncology Group experience, *J Clin Oncol* **13** (1995), 1557–1563.

[25] H.J. Burstein and E.P. Winer, Reproductive Issues, in: *Diseases of the Breast*, 2nd ed., J.R. Harris, M.E. Lippman, M. Morrow and C.K. Osborne, eds, Philadelphia, Lippincott Williams & Wilkins; 2000, pp. 1052–1053.

[26] C.L. Shapiro, J. Manola and M. Leboff, Ovarian failure after adjuvant chemotherapy is associated with rapid bone loss in women with early-stage breast cancer, *J Clin Oncol* **19** (2001), 3306–3311.

[27] P.F. Bruning, M.J. Pit, M. de Long-Bakker et al., Bone mineral density after adjuvant chemotherapy for premenopausal breast cancer, *Br J Cancer* **61** (1990), 308–310.

[28] N. Tchen, F.P. Downie, M. Theriault et al., Cognitive changes and menopausal symptoms in women receiving adjuvant chemotherapy for breast cancer: A matched cohort study, *Proc ASCO* **20** (2001), 110.

[29] I. Tannock, N. Tchen, H. Juffs et al., Fatigue, menopausal symptoms and cognitive dysfunction associated with adjuvant chemotherapy: First year results of a large prospective controlled study, *Breast Cancer Research and Treatment* **76**(1) (2002), S138 (abstract).

[30] C. Brezden, K. Phillips, M. Abdolell et al., Cognitive function in breast cancer patients receiving adjuvant chemotherapy, *J Clin Oncol* **18** (2000), 2695–2701.

[31] T.A. Ahles, A.J. Saykin, C.T. Furstenberg et al., Neuropsychologic impact of standard-dose systemic chemotherapy in long-term survivors of breast cancer and lymphoma, *J Clin Oncol* **20**(2) (2002), 485–493.

[32] S. Schagen, F. Van Dam, M. Muller et al., Cognitive deficits after postoperative adjuvant chemotherapy for breast carcinoma, *Cancer* **85** (1999), 640–650.

[33] F.S. Van Dam, S.B. Schagen, M.J. Muller et al., Impairment of cognitive function in women receiving adjuvant treatment for high-risk breast cancer: high-dose versus standard-dose chemotherapy, *J Natl Cancer Inst* **90** (1998), 210–218.

[34] S.B. Schagen, M.J. Muller, W. Boogerd et al., Late effects of adjuvant chemotherapy on cognitive function: a follow-up study in breast cancer patients, *Annals of Oncology* **13** (2002), 1387–1397.

[35] R. Yancik, M. Wesley, L. Ries et al., Effect of age and comorbidity in postmenopausal breast cancer patients aged 55 years and older, *JAMA* **285** (2001), 885–892.

[36] Satariano, 1994.

[37] S. Rajagopal, P. Goodman and I. Tannock, Adjuvant chemotherapy for breast cancer: Discordance between physicians' perception of benefit and the results of clinical trials, *J Clin Oncol* **12** (1994), 1296–1304.

[38] P.M. Ravdin, I.A. Siminoff and J.A. Harvey, Survey of breast cancer patients concerning their knowledge and expectations of adjuvant therapy, *J Clin Oncol* **16** (1998), 515–521.

[39] C. Lindley, S. Vasa, W. Sawyer et al., Quality of life and preferences for treatment following systemic adjuvant therapy for early-stage breast cancer, *J Clin Oncol* **16** (1998), 1380–1387.

[40] Levine, 1992.

[41] P.M. Ravdin, L.A. Siminoff, G.J. Davis et al., Computer program to assist in making decisions about adjuvant therapy for women with early breast cancer, *J Clin Oncol* **19** (2001), 980–991.

Breast Disease 21 (2004) 41–46
IOS Press

Breast Cancer in the Information Age: A Review of Recent Developments

Paul R. Helft*

Department of Medicine, Division of Hematology/Oncology, Regenstrief Institute for Health Care, and Indiana University Center for Bioethics, Indiana University, Indianapolis, IN, USA

Abstract. Between 50 and 100 million Americans have used the Internet to obtain health information. Breast cancer is one of the most common diagnoses sought online, and breast oncologists are likely to encounter more and more patients who have used the Internet. The effects that this is having on patients and on the clinical encounter in oncology are unclear. Here, the author reviews recent research about the growing importance of online health information and the small amount of literature on breast cancer and the Internet. Other recent developments, such as efforts to recruit patients to clinical trials via the Internet and online support groups for cancer patients, also are reviewed. Finally, the author offers his views on how best to manage patients' growing interest in Internet information.

INTRODUCTION

More and more Americans are turning the Internet to obtain health information. The best estimates are that between 50 and 100 million Americans have sought health information on the Internet [1,2]. On an average day, 5.5 million Americans look up health information online [2]. When the National Library of Medicine created public Medline access in 1997, the number of "hits" went from 7 million in 1996 to 120 million in 1997, with 30% of users coming from the general public [3]. These numbers are growing rapidly each year.

There is emerging evidence that the Internet will play a crucial role in health care. Eleven million Americans who helped a loved one deal with an illness in the past two years say their use of the Internet played a crucial or important role in their aid to another person [2]. More than 4 million Americans say the Internet helped them cope with their own struggle with a major illness in the past two years [4]. More than one-half of all those who have used the Internet to access health information

report that it has improved the way they obtain health information. Almost one-half (41%) of users report that the information they found affected a health care decision [2].

Oncologists on the front lines of cancer care know all too well that patients' use of the Internet is an important phenomenon, and stories abound about patients who show up for their appointment armed with sheaths of Internet downloads [5–7]. Since breast cancer is among the most common health topics sought on the Internet [8], breast oncologists will more and more commonly be asked to help patients sort through the mountains of information (and misinformation) available on the World Wide Web. In this article, I will review the intersection of breast cancer and the Internet, as well as the implications that patients' access to information is likely to have for cancer care in general and breast cancer patients in particular.

THE INTERNET AND CANCER

Although cancer patients clearly are using the Internet in great numbers to obtain information about their disease, we know very little about the effects this unprecedented access to information is having on the clinical encounter in oncology. In North America, the best

---

*Address for correspondence: Paul R. Helft, MD, Division of Hematology/Oncology, 535 Barnhill Drive, RT 473, Indianapolis, IN 46202, USA. Tel.: +1 317 278 6942; Fax: +1 317 278 0079; E-mail: phelft@iupui.edu.

estimates of the proportion of cancer patients using the Internet range from 6% in a Veterans Administration hospital setting [9] to 50% in an urban referral center in Canada [10]. Average estimates of the proportion of cancer patients seeking information online fall in the 30% range [9,11–13].

Early information suggests that patients' use of the Internet to obtain cancer information is influential. In one study, almost 30% of cancer patients who searched the Internet requested specific treatments, and 6% declined the treatments recommended by their oncologists [10]. In another recent survey, American oncologists reported that Internet information could make patients more hopeful, more anxious, more confused, and more knowledgeable [13].

CANCER INFORMATION ON THE INTERNET

Many authors have raised concerns about the hazards of Internet use by patients. Most of these concerns have been about the quality of Internet information and risks of misinformation [5,6,15–17]. Hard evidence that broad-scale "adverse events" are occurring among patients using the Internet is lacking, however. Researchers at the University of Heidelberg have developed a system to attempt to capture Internet adverse events through online event reporting [17].

Eysenbach and colleagues [16] performed the most comprehensive review of the quality of Internet information studies. In this study, the authors examined 79 separate empirical studies that met eligibility criteria. The major findings from this review were that 70% of the examined studies found that the quality of information available on the Internet was a problem. The 9% of studies that found information to be of high quality tended to employ less rigorous methods. So, while many reputable sources of cancer information exist, significant questions remain about the quality of information patients may encounter online.

Multiple initiatives are attempting to review, improve, and assure the quality of online health information. A recent review of major initiatives categorized these efforts into those that used codes of conduct or ethics for websites, those that offered third-party certification of compliance, and those that used tool-based evaluations of quality. The authors concluded that there are still many gaps in the efforts to assure the quality of online health information [18]. Despite these efforts, given the vastness of the World Wide Web and the fact that the Internet is intrinsically difficult to regulate, the quality of health information is likely to remain a significant issue.

BREAST CANCER AND THE INTERNET

Although breast cancer is one of the most common diagnoses sought on the Internet [8], very little published information examines the intersection of breast cancer and the Internet. Only four published studies examine the quality of Internet breast cancer information, and only one study directly examines breast cancer patients themselves.

The few existing studies concerning the quality of online breast cancer information are mixed in their evaluations. Two studies have found Internet breast cancer information to be lacking in quality. One study, examining the relationship between the quality of information on breast cancer sites and popularity of the sites, suggests that popular and less popular sites do not differ with respect to quality of information. Using well-known benchmarks for quality of Internet information [15,19], only 35% of sites evaluated in this study met criteria for high quality of information [20]. A second study, which reviewed 136 breast cancer sites, found that only 32% of sites identified the credentials of the authors, and only 30% indicated the source of information posted [21]. Two studies have reached relatively positive conclusions about breast cancer information. Berland and colleagues examined the quality of Internet breast cancer information and suggested that the information available is more accurate and more complete that a variety of other common conditions [22]. Another study found that only 5.1% of examined breast cancer web sites were inaccurate [23].

Only one published study has directly examined breast cancer patients themselves. A pilot study from researchers at Columbia University in New York City found that of 188 breast cancer patients studied, 41.5% used the Internet for medical information. In addition, it showed that Internet users had a higher income, were more educated, and were slightly more likely to be white than non-white [24].

INTERNET USES

If approximately one-third of cancer patients are using the Internet to obtain cancer information, how are they finding the information and what are they using the Internet for? Relatively few empirical studies address how cancer patients themselves are actually using the Internet or what effects it might be having on them and their clinical decision making. Besides learning about their diseases in general, patients are probably using the

Internet to find medical professionals and second opinions, research new treatments and treatment options, and find information about clinical trials [7]. In much of my own preliminary work with cancer patients in this area, these topics are mentioned most often by cancer patients who use the Internet to obtain information about their disease (unpublished data).

How do patients search for information?

Most information thus far suggests that patients search for information about their diseases using widely available search engines. A Harris Interactive poll recently found that 52% of online health seekers used a portal or search engine to research a health question [1]. Eysenbach and colleagues did an exploratory study in an artificial environment examining the search strategies of 17 people and found that all used search engines as their main search strategy, and that they tended to examine only the first few links found [25]. These findings have a number of implications, since the widely available search engines use varying algorithms for identifying websites. Some search strategies may thus yield higher or lower percentages of quality information sources.

CLINICAL TRIALS, SUPPORT GROUPS AND THE INTERNET

Two interesting online developments for cancer patients and others are the efforts to inform and recruit patients to clinical trials via the Internet and the growing number of online support groups.

Clinical trials and the Internet

Vast amounts of information about clinical trials are now available on the Internet. Many information sites list resources and specific details about available clinical trials in a given disease and many public and private web sites exists for the sole purpose of helping patients find clinical trials for their diseases. The National Institutes of Health have an important presence on the Internet providing disease-specific information about clinical trials sponsored by the various institutes (www.cancernet.nci.nih.gov). Private organizations have launched such efforts as well. These include such Internet companies as www.emergingmed.com, www.veritasmedicine.com, www.americasdoctor.com, www.acurian.com, and www.centerwatch.com . Given

that only 3–5% of adult cancer patients participate in clinical trials in the United States [26,27], and that some do not participate because they do not know that clinical trials are an option [28], using the Internet to inform patients about clinical trials and to link them directly to appropriate clinical trials is an attractive possibility. I have written elsewhere about my views that the efforts to link patients to clinical trials via the Internet, particularly by private, for-profit companies, raise a number of ethical concerns, including issues of informed consent, protection of vulnerable patient populations, and patient selection [29]. Nearly everyone agrees, however, that recruiting more cancer patients to clinical trials is a worthwhile goal.

Internet support groups

The benefits of support groups for cancer patients are well documented [30–32]. There is emerging evidence that cancer patients are using the Internet and online resources for social support [33–35]. Authors writing in this area describe many advantages of Internet-based support groups, including relative anonymity, the ability to participate in a controlled fashion and despite geographical distance or infirmity, the ability to share the experiences of patients with similar conditions, 24 hours a day availability, and increased participation of men. The growing number of online support groups for patients can take the form of newsgroups (where messages appear as running lists of comments or questions), listservs (which automatically distribute messages in the form of e-mail documents to names on a mailing list), and chat rooms (which provide users the opportunity to communicate in real time through messages posted through instant messaging software to users registered in a given "room"). Lists of well-established cancer online support groups are available [35].

ONCOLOGISTS' VIEW OF INTERNET USE BY CANCER PATIENTS

It is now common, in my experience, to hear oncologists sharing "war stories" of their clinical encounters with Internet-avid patients. Some have even written about the negative effects this is having on their own practice [5,6]. I would like to summarize here some recent work done in an effort to assess oncologists' views of Internet use by cancer patients more broadly, as well as the effects it may be having on the practice of oncology. The full details of this study are available elsewhere [13].

In this study, a brief mail survey was sent to a systematic sample of 5% of United States medical oncologists and hematologist/oncologists listed in the membership directory of the American Society of Clinical Oncology. The overall response rate was 46.2%. Oncologists' median estimate of the proportion of their patients using the Internet to obtain cancer information was 30%, and they estimated that about one third of these patients brought Internet information to discuss in a clinic visit. Subjects responded that, on average, 10 minutes were added to each patient encounter in which Internet information was discussed. Responding oncologists reported that use of the Internet had the ability simultaneously to make patients more hopeful, confused, anxious, and knowledgeable. Forty-four percent of responding oncologists reported that they sometimes or rarely had difficulty discussing Internet information and only 9% of subjects reported that they sometimes or always felt threatened when patients brought Internet information to discuss. Those who had difficulty discussing Internet information were more likely to report feeling threatened. In narrative responses, oncologists reported both positive and negative effects of Internet use by patients.

What was fairly clear from this study was that, according to practicing medical oncologists, a significant proportion of cancer patients appears to be using the Internet to obtain cancer information, and that oncologists viewed Internet information as having both positive and negative effects on the clinical encounter. This study raises a number of questions about the best way of "managing" patients' interest in and use of the Internet.

THE INTERNET AND THE ONCOLOGIST-PATIENT RELATIONSHIP

Oncologists who care for cancer patients have a privileged position and often care for patients during the most difficult period of their lives. Cancer decision-making has a number of unique properties, also, which render the process of reaching therapeutic decisions very complex. These include the life-threatening nature of malignant disease, the psychosocial weight of the cancer diagnosis, the acuity of the decisions, and the ponderous trade-offs between the risks and benefits of what are commonly arduous treatments. This has never been more true than in the case of the adjuvant therapy for breast cancer, which is actively in evolu-

tion and relies on careful tailoring of treatment recommendations to individual patients and disease characteristics [36–38]. Many patients obviously recognize the complexity of the decision-making and turn to the Internet for further information.

Given the paucity of empirical information about the effects of Internet cancer information on the clinical care of cancer patients, how should practicing oncologists deal with patients who use the Internet? I would make two recommendations based on personal and collective experience, and the small but growing literature in this area.

Accept patients' use of the Internet

Patients' use of the Internet is only going to grow. Early evidence from my own work in this area suggests that one of the sources of resistance to Internet use by cancer patients may be the perceived threat to authority posed by patients' access to information. It is true that in many ways patients have equal access to information as their physicians. I have heard many stories of oncologists who learned of new clinical trials and options for treatment from their patients, as often the patients have more focused time to look for information on the Internet than their busy oncologists do. For most patients, information-seeking about their illness represents a powerful coping mechanism, and there are many reasons to support the behavior.

The difficulty in this has not escaped me, and poses three significant problems. First, patients will inevitably encounter misinformation on the Internet. This should be viewed as an opportunity to correct misunderstandings and to point patients to quality sources of information. It is helpful to spend a bit of time reviewing Internet sources of cancer information, and to become familiar with websites of high quality, and even to generate a printed list of sites which one could recommend as being of high quality.

Second, in my view, the greatest difficulty posed by Internet information is not quality, but individualization. I find that patients commonly have more trouble identifying which information applies to their specific case than identifying quality information. Oncologists are perfectly suited to correct such misunderstandings, and, indeed, such discussions can actually strengthen rapport and trust with between patients and oncologists.

Third, I commonly hear the objection that practicing oncologists do not have time to sort through hundreds of web pages with patients. My own research suggests that for busy oncologists in practices where a high proportion of patients is using the Internet and bringing information to discuss during their clinical encounters, this activity can pose a significant time burden. Nevertheless, several suggestions culled from clever colleagues can help busy practicing oncologists deal with this situation.

One strategy is to ask patients to boil down their questions to the two or three issues raised by Internet information that they feel are most important to be answered; this strategy helps to focus the discussion on issues raised by Internet information which are most important to patients. A second strategy, when faced with patients with large stacks of downloaded information about which an opinion is desired, is to ask permission to take the stack of papers and to review it later, with a commitment to discuss the information in a second clinical encounter. A related strategy I have seen used by some oncologists is to offer to read the information and to schedule a follow-up telephone conversation to answer questions or concerns.

Create positive clinical encounters using patients' interest in Internet information

The mail survey study summarized above [13] included a write-in question in which oncologists were asked to describe a patient encounter that summarized the impact of Internet information on their practice. Many responding oncologists wrote enlightening anecdotes in response to this. One message was that discussions with patients concerning Internet information can be used to strengthen the oncologist-patient relationship. For example, patients occasionally appear to place more belief in information they read on the Internet than in the things their oncologists tell them. Several responders to our survey noted that the time spent explaining in a non-threatening (and non-threatened) way why many things found on the Internet were not true or did not apply to an individual's case, led to very positive discussions, and helped to foster trust on the part of patients. Others cited examples in which patients identified an appropriate clinical trial or new treatment not offered by the oncologist. Although this is a potentially awkward situation, open acceptance of such inquiry, including offers to facilitate second opinions and refer patients to institutions offering clinical trials, can actually lead to positive feelings on the part of patients.

CONCLUSION

The Internet is changing many aspects of our lives in profound ways we are only beginning to understand. It is likely to be having a profound and lasting impact on medical care, including the complex care of cancer patients. I am personally very positive with respect to the changes the Internet is likely to bring to cancer care: more informed patients, more rapid dissemination of new information, and the potential to expand access to clinical trials. There is nothing more pleasing to me as a practicing oncologist than sitting down with a well-informed, thoughtful patient who has read as much about their disease as I have, and having a deep discussion of the risks and benefits of treatment. When this happens, it represents a model of cancer care and, indeed, of informed consent itself.

REFERENCES

[1] H. Taylor and R. Leitman, eHealth traffic critically dependent on search engines and portals, See http://www.Harrisinteractive.Com/news/newsletters/healthnews/hi_healthcarenews2001vol1_iss13.Pdf. Accessed January 27, 2003.

[2] Pew Research Center, The online health care revolution: How the web helps Americans take better care of themselves. See http://www.pewinternet.org/reports/toc.asp?Report=26. Accessed January 27, 2003.

[3] National Library of Medicine. National Library of Medicine to work with public libraries to help consumers find answers to medical questions. See http://www.Nlm.Nih.Gov/news/press_releases/medplus.Html. Accessed January 27, 2003.

[4] Pew Research Center. Use of the Internet at Major Life Moments. See http://www.Pewinternet.Org/reports/reports.Asp?Report=58§ion=reportlevel1&field=level1id&id=256. Accessed May 6, 2002.

[5] M. Markman, Cancer and the internet: The good, the bad, and the very ugly, *Curr Oncol Rep* **3** (2001), 77–78.

[6] M. Markman, Cancer information and the Internet: Benefits and risks, *Cleve Clin J Med* **65** (1998), 274–276.

[7] G. Kolata, Web research transforms visit to the doctor, *New York Times* (2000), A1,A6.

[8] Lacroix E-M. MEDLINEplus. See http://www.Nlm.Nih.Gov/pubs/staffpubs/lo/medlineplus/sld013.Htm. Accessed January 27, 2003.

[9] J.M. Metz, P. Devine, A. DeNittis et al., Utilization of the Internet by oncology patients to obtain cancer related information, *Proc ASCO* (2001), Abstract 1575.

[10] X. Chen and L.L. Siu, Impact of the media and the Internet on oncology: Survey of cancer patients and oncologists in Canada, *J Clin Oncol* **19** (20010, 4291–4297.

[11] S. Yakren, W. Shi, H. Thaler et al., Use of Internet and other information resources among adult cancer patients and their companions, *Proc ASCO* (2001), Abstract 1589.

[12] P.R. Helft, F. Hlubocky, E.J. Gordon, M.J. Ratain and C.K. Daugherty, Hope and the media in advanced cancer patients, *Proc ASCO* (2000), Abstract 2497.

[13] P.R. Helft, F. Hlubocky and C.K. Daugherty, American oncologists' views of internet use by cancer patients: A mail survey of American Society of Clinical Oncology members, *J Clin Oncol* (2003), 21.

[14] W.M. Silberg, G.D. Lundberg and R.A. Musacchio, Assessing, controlling, and assuring the quality of medical information on the Internet: Caveant lector et viewor–let the reader and viewer beware, *JAMA* **277** (1997), 1244–1245.

[15] S.D. McLeod, The quality of medical information on the Internet. A new public health concern, *Arch Ophthalmol* **116** (1998), 1663–1665.

[16] G. Eysenbach, J. Powell, O. Kuss and E.R. Sa, Empirical studies assessing the quality of health information for consumers on the World Wide Web: A systematic review, *JAMA* **287** (2002), 2691–2700.

[17] Database of adverse events related to the Internet (DAERI). See http://www.Medcertain.Org/daeri/. Accessed January 20, 2003.

[18] A. Risk and J. Dzenowagis, Review of Internet health information quality initiatives, *J Med Internet Res* (2001), 3:e28.

[19] Health on the Net Foundation. HON code of conduct (Honcode) for medical and health websites: Principles. See http://www.hon.ch/HONcode/Conduct.html. Accessed January 30, 2003.

[20] F. Meric, E.V. Bernstam, N.Q. Mirza et al., Breast cancer on the World Wide Web: Cross sectional survey of quality of information and popularity of websites, *BMJ* **324** (2002), 577–581.

[21] L. Hoffman-Goetz and J.N. Clarke, Quality of breast cancer sites on the World Wide Web, *Can J Pub Health* **91** (2000), 281–284.

[22] G.K. Berland, M.N. Elliott, L.S. Morales et al., Health information on the Internet: Accessibility, quality, and readability in English and Spanish, *JAMA* **285** (2001), 2612–2621.

[23] J. Shon and M.A. Musen, The low availability of meta-data elements for evaluating the quality of medical information on the World Wide Web, *Proc AMIA Symp* (1999), 945–949.

[24] J. Fogel, S.M. Albert, F. Schnabel, B.A. Ditkoff and A.I. Neugut, Use of the Internet by women with breast cancer, *J Med Internet Res* (2002), 4:e9.

[25] G. Eysenbach, How do consumers search for and appraise health information on the world wide web? Qualitative study using focus groups, usability tests, and in-depth interviews, *BMJ* **324** (2002), 573–577.

[26] P.N. Lara, Jr., R. Higdon, N. Lim et al., Prospective evaluation of cancer clinical trial accrual patterns: Identifying potential barriers to enrollment, *J Clin Oncol* **19** (2001), 1728–1733.

[27] A.B. Benson, J.P. Pregler, J.A. Bean et al., Oncologists' reluctance to accrue patients onto clinical trials: An Illinois cancer center study, *J Clin Oncol* **9** (1991), 2067–2075.

[28] H. Taylor and R. Leitman, Harris Interactive. Misconceptions and lack of awareness greatly reduce recruitment for cancer clinical trials. See http://www.harrisinteractive.com/news/newsletters/healthnews/HL HealthCareNews2001VolL iss3.pdf. Accessed January 27, 2003.

[29] P.R. Helft, Clinical trials information and recruitment on the internet: Technological breakthrough or ethical nightmare? *Clinical Researcher* **1** (2001), 31–34.

[30] D.F. Cella and S.B. Yellen, Cancer support groups: The state of the art, *Cancer Pract* **1** (1993), 56–61.

[31] M.J. Galinsky and J.H. Schopler, Negative experiences in support groups, *Soc Work Health Care* **20** (1994), 77–95.

[32] N. Samarel and J. Fawcett, Enhancing adaptation to breast cancer: The addition of coaching to support groups, *Oncol Nurs Forum* **19** (1992), 591–596.

[33] P. Klemm, K. Reppert and L. Visich, A nontraditional cancer support group, *The Internet. Computers in Nursing* **16** (1998), 31–36.

[34] S.P. LaCoursiere, A theory of online social support, *Advances in Nursing Science* **24** (2001), 60–77.

[35] S.D. Martin and K.B. Youngren, The virtual community: Helping patients use Internet support groups, *Home Healthcare Nurse* **18** (2000), 333–335.

[36] C.L. Loprinzi and S.D. Thome, Understanding the utility of adjuvant systemic therapy for primary breast cancer, *J Clin Oncol* **19** (2001), 972–979.

[37] A. Goldhirsch, J.H. Glick, R.D. Gelber, A.S. Coates and H.J. Senn, Meeting highlights: International consensus panel on the treatment of primary breast cancer. Seventh international conference on adjuvant therapy of primary breast cancer, *J Clin Oncol* **19** (2001), 3817–3827.

[38] A.R. Tan and S.M. Swain, Adjuvant chemotherapy for breast cancer: An update, *Semin Oncol* **28** (2001), 359–376.

Breast Disease 21 (2004) 47–54
IOS Press

Rational Surveillance Programs for Early Stage Breast Cancer Patients After Primary Treatment

Joseph A. Mollick and Robert W. Carlson*
Department of Medicine, Division of Medical Oncology, Stanford University, Stanford, CA 94305, USA

Abstract. The majority of women with early stage breast cancers are successfully treated with surgery, radiation therapy and adjuvant systemic therapy. However, 30% of all Stage I and Stage II patients can be expected to experience a relapse. The belief that early detection of recurrences can lead to an increase in survival has been used to justify intensive follow-up regimens following primary treatment of patients with early stage disease. However, the vast majority of data support a program of scheduled surveillance visits and demonstrate that a comprehensive history and physical examination is as efficacious as programs utilizing intensive testing and imaging procedures in the asymptomatic patient. Screening mammography to detect ipsilateral in-breast recurrence or a new primary cancer in the contralateral breast is the only imaging study that is recommended for routine surveillance. Knowledge of the natural history of breast cancer, risk factors for relapse, and the symptoms and physical findings commonly associated with recurrence are central to efficiently and effectively monitoring this cohort of women in clinical practice.

POTENTIAL BIASES IN STUDIES OF THE EARLY DETECTION OF BREAST CANCER RECURRENCE

Surveillance programs following primary treatment are based on the belief that early detection and treatment of recurrence offers a better chance of cure, improved survival or enhanced quality of life. A number of studies, both retrospective and prospective, have evaluated the use of clinic visits, serum tests and imaging procedures to assess their value in terms of survival, economics and quality of life.

Several forms of potential bias impact the reliability of studies using survival as an endpoint for surveillance protocols. The first is lead-time bias and refers to the analysis of the time interval between the discovery of recurrence by a clinical test in an asymptomatic patient and the time a patient would have brought the recur-

rence to the attention of her physician. Even if the subsequent treatment has no impact on patient outcome, early detection of recurrence will be associated with an increase in survival from date of detection, even though mortality (date of death) is not changed. The second bias is the length bias, and refers to the increased number of opportunities to diagnose slowly growing tumors by tests performed at regular, defined intervals. This is in contrast to faster growing, more aggressive tumors that appear in between the testing intervals that quickly cause symptoms and are brought to the attention of the doctor by the patient. Thus, the biologic characteristics of tumors diagnosed by surveillance procedures are likely to be more biologically favorable than tumors diagnosed in the intervals between surveillance visits. Both lead-time bias and length-bias may make it appear that more intensive surveillance programs lead to increased duration of survival from time of recurrence, when in fact they may provide no benefit to survival overall.

Other bias types are frequently encountered in studies of surveillance programs. For example, screening tests routinely used in surveillance programs most of-

*Corresponding author: Robert W. Carlson, M.D., Division of Oncology, Stanford University Medical Center, 1000 Welch Road, Suite 202, Palo Alto, CA 94304, USA. Tel.: +1 650 725 6457; Fax: +1 650 725 8222; E-mail: rcarlson@stanford.edu.

ten find lesions at biologically favorable sites. Physical exams find local or regional recurrences, chest radiographs find early effusions or nodules. By contrast, unfavorable visceral or central nervous system recurrences are infrequently detected by serum chemistries and more often present with symptoms. Thus, simply by detecting asymptomatic disease in favorable sites, surveillance programs may appear to benefit overall survival compared to patients who present with symptomatic disease at unfavorable sites.

The biases inherent in many surveillance studies may be partially overcome by study designs that include randomized comparison groups (and that utilize survival) from the date of initial diagnosis as the primary endpoint rather than from date of detection of first recurrence.

DETECTION OF FIRST RECURRENCE

One of the goals of any surveillance program is to reveal a recurrence before it presents as symptoms. An early retrospective study using a database of 400 patients demonstrated that 73% of recurrences were found by the patients in between follow-up visits [1]. Only 27% of first recurrences were found specifically as a result of follow-up surveillance. There was no difference in the overall survival of the two groups of patients after therapy was instituted. Other similarly designed studies have arrived at similar conclusions [2,3]. One of the largest of these retrospective analyses used the ECOG database of breast cancer patients enrolled in adjuvant clinical trials [4]. Of 208 evaluable patients with relapse, 54% were brought to the attention of the physician by the patient. Physical examination of the asymptomatic patient by the physician identified an additional 19% of the recurrences. The remainder of the recurrences, approximately 25%, were detected in asymptomatic patients by a combination of blood chemistries, bone scans, chest x-rays and mammograms.

An analysis of the annual hazard of recurrence rates in patients entered onto 7 large ECOG trials provided quantitative rates of relapse in breast cancer patients [5]. The results of this analysis demonstrated that the annual hazard of recurrence was greatest for the interval between years 1 and 2 after surgery, peaking at 13%. The hazard rate then decreased until year 5. Beyond 5 years, the annual hazard rate for recurrence declined slowly and averaged about 4.3% each year. These data emphasize that the hazard of recurrence is not constant throughout the first 10 years of follow-up, and the haz-

ard of recurrence peaks between 1 and 2 years following surgery. Thus, the first years following diagnosis are a particularly high-risk period, justifying more frequent follow-up visits during this time period. The early period of follow-up is also an excellent time to enroll patients on risk reduction trials or early detection of recurrence trials. Even patients beyond 5 years of follow-up have measurable relapse rates and thus are candidates for risk reduction trials looking at novel agents. For women enrolled on trials with disease free survival (DFS) or disease free interval (DFI) as an endpoint, systematic follow-up is critical to document disease recurrence. In this setting, the schedule of follow-up may be altered to achieve the goals of the specific clinical trial.

RANDOMIZED TRIALS ASSESSING SURVEILLANCE

Two randomized trials have compared the use of minimal versus more intensive surveillance in women following primary treatment for breast cancer. The Gruppo Interdisciplinare perla Valutazione degli Interventi in Oncologia (GIVIO) investigators reported a multi-institutional trial of 1320 women with Stage I, II or III breast cancer [6]. Women were randomized to intensive surveillance including physician assessments, bone scans, liver echography, chest x-ray, mammography, serum alkaline phosphatase, and γ-glutyltranspeptidase or to a control regimen that included the physician assessments and mammography only. At a median of 71 months of follow-up, there were no differences between the surveillance groups in terms of time to detection of recurrence, survival, or health related quality of life.

A second study of intensive surveillance involved 1,243 women with surgically treated breast cancer [7]. The patients were randomized to physician assessment plus annual mammography with or without routine chest radiographs and bone scans. Breast cancer recurrences were detected earlier in the intensive surveillance group. However, cumulative mortality at 10 years in the intensive surveillance group was 34.8% versus 31.5% in the clinical follow-up group (hazard ration, 1.05; 95% confidence interval 0.87–1.26) [8].

IN-BREAST RECURRENCE FOLLOWING BREAST CONSERVATION

In-breast recurrences following breast conservation are an important exception where early detection and treatment of recurrence appears to provide benefit. Local recurrences are most often discovered by the examining physician, and most frequently in asymptomatic patients. In this subcategory of women with asymptomatic local recurrences, 5-year survival rates of approximately 50% are observed [9].

EMOTIONAL WELL BEING AND QUALITY OF LIFE

One powerful argument for a regimented, routine surveillance strategy is that it provides a framework to explain to patients. Patients find this set schedule for early detection of recurrence by history and physical examination reassuring. Surveys of patient preferences on follow-up practices are quite revealing and indicate the need for patient education during the period of secondary surveillance. In a survey of a breast cancer clinic in North Carolina, only one-third of patients recognized the value of history taking in detecting recurrence and only two-thirds recognized the value of a physical examination [10]. Laboratory data and imaging procedures were rated higher than history taking in detecting recurrences. Ninety-two percent of patients believed that early detection of recurrence improved long-term outlook, potential for cure or chance of response to subsequent therapy. Knowledge of the value and limitations of testing was not related to patient educational level.

More insights emerged in the GIVO trial [6]. In this trial, quality-of-life and treatment-preference questionnaires were completed by patients at 6 months, 1, 2 and 5 years. The data from this trial suggest that various dimensions of quality of life measures did not differ between the intensive testing arm and the control arm. Once again, diagnostic tests were highly valued by the majority of patients (70%) at each of the time points tested. This preference to be followed with clinical testing was independent of the treatment arm that they were enrolled in and was independent of the presence of symptoms.

Routine surveillance visits provide the opportunity to identify and initiate interventions relating to late sequele of treatment or the disease process itself. Depression, sexual dysfunction and menopausal symptoms are common in the post-treatment breast cancer population and effective interventions are often available. Simply being reassured that she remains "cancer-free" by her physician may speed a woman's return to normal social functioning and enhance self-esteem.

THE EFFECT OF TUMOR CHARACTERISTICS AND TREATMENT HISTORY ON THE SITES OF RELAPSE

Early adjuvant trials attempted to correlate the frequency of relapse at various sites and the administration of post-operative chemotherapy [3,11,12]. These early studies generally concluded that relapse was less frequently found in patients given adjuvant chemotherapy, but no substantial differences in patterns of relapse were found. Tumors that express the estrogen receptor are more likely to relapse in visceral organs than those that lack this receptor [13,14]. Lobular carcinomas are known to have a biological predisposition to recur on serosal surfaces such as the peritoneum and leptomeninges [15,16]. Recent data from gene profiling experiments on breast cancer suggest that the metastatic potential of tumors may be determined early in the natural history of the disease. This is in contra-distinction from the hypothesis that metastases represent an evolution of the primary tumor to take on this characteristic [17–20]. If site-specific metastases are a function of cell surface adhesion molecules or proteinases, then it is possible that gene profiling studies may be able to predict not just relapse, but also site of relapse.

ASSOCIATION OF METASTASES WITH SYMPTOMS

Early detection of recurrent breast cancer depends on knowledge of the symptoms that typically herald recurrent disease. Retrospective and prospective studies indicate that 50% to 70% of patients will bring symptoms to the attention of their physician that will lead to the diagnosis of recurrent breast cancer. However, local regional recurrences are more often discovered by physician assessment than is distant disease. For example, in one study, 60% of patients with local-regional recurrences were found by physician examination, as opposed to distant metastases that more often present with patient complaints [21]. Thus, a productive surveillance clinic visit should include a comprehensive review of systems that interrogates symptoms relating to the most common sites of recurrent disease.

ASSESSMENT OF THE SYMPTOMATIC PATIENT

Bony recurrences

Bone-only recurrences are a common clinical scenario and have also been intensively studied. Bone pain is the most common symptom suggestive of bone lesions. However, the specificity of bone scintigraphy is low, and often bone scan abnormalities are indicative of benign disease. The number of abnormalities on a bone scan can be used to aid in this distinction. For example, in one series a single bone scan abnormality eventually lead to the diagnosis of metastatic disease in 11% of patients, whereas two abnormalities lead to this diagnosis in 24%. The pelvis and sternum were the sites most specific for recurrent disease, at 50% and 33%, respectively [22]. Follow-up bone scans were also useful in making the distinction between metastases and benign disease. In the absence of new therapy, bone metastases nearly always become more intense, where as benign abnormalities remain unchanged or resolve [22]. Plain bone radiographs are useful for distinguishing metastatic from benign disease and should always be performed on the sites of a newly positive bone scan. Magnetic Resonance Imaging (MRI) is a useful test to distinguish abnormalities in the spine. The spine is a common site of relapse, but also a site of benign abnormalities on a bone scan. An MRI may help to distinguish between compression fractures secondary to tumor or osteoporosis. However, false positive MRI scans in the spine are not uncommon. PET scans may have a role in evaluating bone pain complaints in breast cancer surveillance. In a small series of 12 patients, Wahl et al. reported that PET correctly identified 10/10 bone metastases [23,24].

Liver recurrences

Liver involvement with cancer in general is heralded by non-specific complaints of anorexia, malaise, weight loss and abdominal pain. Jaundice and liver enzyme abnormalities are late and uncommon first signs of relapse in the liver. Suspected liver involvement is best evaluated with a contrast-enhanced abdominal CT scan. Incidental findings in the liver are common, and most often represent hemangiomas. As the liver is uncommonly a solitary site of relapse, isolated findings in the liver should be interpreted with caution, and a full restaging evaluation with a chest and pelvic CT scan and bone scan should also be performed.

Pulmonary recurrences

Pulmonary metastases frequently present with cough, shortness of breath or chest pain. If symptomatic, lung abnormalities are most often visible on a plain chest radiograph. Chest CT scans are far more sensitive than chest radiographs and should be performed if the radiographs are uninformative. As with the liver, the lungs are rarely the site of a solitary recurrence, and any evidence of recurrent disease in the lungs should be evaluated with a full restaging evaluation. Isolated lung findings, including pleural effusions, should be pursued for a definitive histologic diagnosis. Pleural effusions secondary to breast cancer are almost always cytologically positive.

Central nervous system recurrences

Symptoms suggestive of central nervous system involvement include headaches, neck pain, cord compression, cranial nerve findings or motor or sensory deficits. Careful attention should be paid to complaints of radicular pain, parathesias and weakness in the ipsilateral arm and shoulder as these symptoms can indicate an axillary or brachial plexus relapse. As with pulmonary and hepatic involvement, isolated relapse in the central nervous system is rare, and should always be interpreted in the context of a complete restaging evaluation to look for other sites of involvement. Tissue biopsy to prove recurrence is always preferred, and can be carried out on a non-CNS site more easily. No one site of CNS involvement is typical of breast cancer. The tumors can be parenchymal, leptomeningeal, or dural-based with extension. MRI scans are the most sensitive imaging modality of the central nervous system and can detect masses less than 1 cm in size.

CIRCULATING TUMOR MARKERS AND INVESTIGATIONAL APPROACHES TO SURVEILLANCE

The lack of clinical benefit shown in more intensive surveillance protocols has led to the attempts to develop less invasive, more cost-effective means of detecting disease recurrence. A number of circulating tumor antigens have been found to be elevated in some breast cancer patients, and have been studied for detection of recurrence. These antigens include carcinoembryonic antigen (CEA), tissue polypepide antigen (TPA) and MUC-1 (a mucin-like, membrane glycoprotein). MUC-1 is a cell surface molecule that undergoes aberrant glycosolation during malignant transformation. ELISA assays are used to measure MUC-1 in the serum. Depending upon the assay system used, circulating MUC-1 is measured as CA15-3 or CA27.29. Breast cancer tumor markers have significant limitations [25]. A marker's utility depends on test characteristics, sensitivity, specificity and assay variability. In addition, the usefulness of these tests is dependent upon the efficacy of therapy that will be prompted by positive test results. For example, if poorly effective therapy exists for a tumor, the serum markers may be useful for disease bulk and prognosis, but non-informative for predicting therapeutic response or benefit.

A recent study retrospectively compared the sensitivity of CA15-3 and CA27.29, and concluded that the CA27.29 test is more sensitive [26]. One of the more recent and better executed studies that revisited the utility of these tumor markers was reported in 1997. Chan and colleagues used a competitive binding RIA with the anti-MUC1 monoclonal antibody, B27.29 [27]. They examined 166 treated patients diagnosed with stage II and III disease. All patients had no evidence of disease at the beginning of the study. With a mean of 13 months follow-up, 18 recurrences were detected. The CA27.29 test had a sensitivity of 57.7%, a specificity of 97.9%, and a positive predictive value of 83.3%. The CA27.29 assay was equally sensitive in local-regional and distant recurrence (62% versus 55%). The lead-time provided by a positive test result was longer in distant recurrence compared to local-regional recurrence (6.7 vs. 2.3 months). Because of the study design, the actual lead times are likely to be twice as long as reported. The assay was 100% sensitive and specific in detecting bone metastases in patients with bone pain complaints.

More recent reports examined the use of FDG-PET imaging in patients with elevated CA15-3 or CEA levels and equivocal or negative routine imaging studies to define the site of relapse [28]. Thirty patients were examined in whom routine imaging studies could not unequivocally establish the diagnosis. The final diagnosis of recurrent breast cancer was established by tissue biopsy. FDG-PET accurately detected 35/38 sites in 25/28 patients with recurrence. The sensitivity of 96%, a combination of the sensitivity of the tumor marker and the PET scan, suggests PET scans may be useful as a single imaging modality to investigate the significance of a positive tumor marker test. Additional studies with larger patient numbers will be required to better define the utility of PET scanning, with or without tumor markers, in surveillance testing. As with other tumor markers studies, endpoints with overall survival and quality of life will have to be included in such studies.

The sensitivity of both CA15-3 and CA27.29 tests raises the question of how to respond to elevated test results. No study has yet demonstrated an advantage to initiation of therapy based upon an elevated or rising CA15-3 or CA27.29 in the surveillance population. Treatment begun with increasing marker levels may extend the disease symptom-free interval [29]. Based upon the available data, tumor markers are not recommended for routine breast cancer surveillance nor is an elevated or rising tumor marker considered sufficient for the diagnosis of recurrent disease. The ASCO Clinical Practice Guideline recommendations for the use of CA15-3 and CA27.29 in surveillance of breast cancer patients has not changed since these tests were developed. The 2000 guidelines concluded that without substantial changes in therapy options, and without a demonstration of improved survival, decreased toxicity, increased quality of life, or superior cost-effectiveness that the tests could not be recommended [30].

BREAST CANCER SURVEILLANCE: WHO DOES THE SURVEYING?

Several studies have examined the outcomes of women followed by specialists and generalists. In general, such studies have shown that women fair equally well when follow by specialists, internists, or family physicians, after completion of all therapy. For example, a British study randomized 296 women to follow-up after primary treatment with a medical oncologist, or a community based general practitioner [31]. Of the small number of relapses in this population thus far, there were no data to suggest that the diagnosis of recurrence was delayed in the group seeing a community physician. When questioned regarding whom should do routine surveillance exams, the specialist and generalist each felt that they were best qualified. A number of patient surveys fail to provide an overriding theme, but generally the patients prefer specialists, at least for several years after treatment [32].

ADHERENCE TO PUBLISHED TREATMENT GUIDELINES

Few studies have assessed the actual frequency at which radiographic and laboratory tests are ordered during the surveillance of women following treatment for early stage breast cancer. In one study, physician self-reporting of surveillance testing was studied focusing on postmenopausal women with early stage breast cancer. One study found medical oncologist more

Table 1
Recommended surveillance programs following primary treatment of early breast cancer

Professional organization	History and physical examination	Mammography, conserved breast	Mammography contralateral breast	Test Recommended		
				Tumor markers, chemistries, blood count	Bone scans	Radiographs, CT/MRI or PET scans
ASCO breast cancer surveillance guideline [34]	Every 3 to 6 months for 3 years; Every 6 to 12 months for 2 years; Annually beyond 5 years	6 months following completion of breast irradiation, then as per contralateral breast	Yearly	No	No	No
NCCN Guideline [35]	Every 4–6 months for 5 years; Annually beyond 5 years	6 months after completion of breast irradiation, then as per contralateral breast	Yearly	No	No	No
Canadian medical association [36]	Frequency individualized; At least every 12 months	Yearly	Yearly	No	No	No
National breast cancer center of Australia [37]	Every 3 months for 1 year; Every 6 months for 4 years; Annually beyond 5 years	6–12 months after completion of breast irradiation, then as per contralateral breast	Yearly	No	No	No
European society of medical oncology [38]	Every 3–6 months for 3 years; Every 6–12 months for 2 years; Annually beyond 5 years	Every 1–2 years	Every 1–2 years	No	No	No

likely to adopt an intensive practice style compared to radiation oncologists or surgeons [33]. Regional variations in practice pattern were observed, with oncologists in the northeast and midwest adopting a more intensive style than those in the west and south. Other provider characteristics such as gender, prior experience and practice type had no effect on surveillance patterns in a multivariate analysis. This study, performed in 1991 may not reflect actual patterns today. However, the wide variations highlight the differences in practice patterns that exist in the United States.

RECOMMENDED GUIDELINES FOR BREAST CANCER SURVEILLANCE

Several professional organizations have produced evidence-based guidelines that provide a framework plan for follow-up surveillance of patients following primary treatment for breast cancer.

The American Society of Clinical Oncology (ASCO) last updated its evidence-based surveillance recommendations for breast cancer in 1998 [34]. The ASCO recommendations regarding test selection and frequency are based upon the identified endpoints of overall survival, disease free survival, quality of life and toxicity reduction. Cost effectiveness is also considered as a secondary endpoint. The guidelines recommend monthly breast self-examinations and annual mammography of the preserved and contralateral breast.

The ASCO guidelines recommend a history and physical examination every 3–6 months for 3 years, then every 6 to 12 months for 2 years. After year 5, routine exams are annual. Specifically, no radiographic imaging (other than mammography), blood chemistries or tumor markers are recommended in the absence of specific symptoms or physical findings.

The 2002 National Cancer Center Network Breast Cancer Treatment Guideline provides recommendations for breast cancer [35]. The NCCN guidelines recommend interval history and physical exams every 4–6 months for 5 years then every 12 months. Mammograms are continued every 12 months in the unaffected breast and every 6 months in the conserved breast, if applicable, for 2 years and then annually thereafter. Women being treated with tamoxifen should receive a pelvic exam every 12 months if the uterus is present. No other routine testing is recommended in the absence of symptoms or physical findings.

Other national and international organizations have provided recommendations for follow-up surveillance following primary treatment of early breast cancer (Table 1). These multiple guidelines are remarkably consistent with each other regarding recommended surveillance procedures.

SUMMARY

Good quality clinical studies to date support a regimented follow-up plan for women treated for early stage breast cancer. However, the regimen includes only a history, physical examination and screening mammography. The data do not support the use one of a number of imaging modalities or blood tests. The current recommendations, endorsed by North American, Australian, and European professional organizations will require modification when the treatment of recurrent breast cancer becomes substantially more efficacious. Without major treatment advances, the recommendations are unlikely to change. Future challenges to the recommended surveillance programs should incorporate a randomized study design and have the power to demonstrate increases in quality of life, symptom-free survival and overall survival.

REFERENCES

[1] A. Zwaveling, G.H. Albers, W. Felthuis and J. Hermans, An evaluation of routine follow-up for detection of breast cancer recurrences, *J Surg Oncol* **34** (1987), 194–197.

[2] T. Broyn and J. Froyen, Evaluation of routine follow-up after surgery for breast carcinoma, *Acta Chir Scand* **148** (1982), 401–404.

[3] D.P. Winchester, S.F. Sener, J.D. Khandekar, M.A. Oviedo, M.P. Cunningham, J.A. Caprini et al., Symptomatology as an indicator of recurrent or metastatic breast cancer, *Cancer* **43** (1979), 956–960.

[4] K.J. Pandya, E.T. McFadden, L.A. Kalish, D.C. Tormey, S.G.t. Taylor and G. Falkson, A retrospective study of earliest indicators of recurrence in patients on Eastern Cooperative Oncology Group adjuvant chemotherapy trials for breast cancer. A preliminary report, *Cancer* **55** (1985), 202–205.

[5] T. Saphner, D.C. Tormey and R. Gray, Annual hazard rates of recurrence for breast cancer after primary therapy, *J Clin Oncol* **14** (1996), 2738–2746.

[6] Impact of follow-up testing on survival and health-related quality of life in breast cancer patients. A multicenter randomized controlled trial. The GIVIO Investigators, *JAMA* **271** (1994), 1587–1592.

[7] M. Rosselli Del Turco, D. Palli, A. Cariddi, S. Ciatto, P. Pacini and V. Distante, Intensive diagnostic follow-up after treatment of primary breast cancer. A randomized trial. National Research Council Project on Breast Cancer follow-up, *JAMA* **271** (1994), 1593–1597.

[8] D. Palli, A. Russo, C. Saieva, S. Ciatto, M. Rosselli Del Turco, V. Distante et al., Intensive vs clinical follow-up after treatment of primary breast cancer: 10-year update of a randomized trial. National Research Council Project on Breast Cancer Follow-up, *JAMA* **281** (1999), 1586.

[9] R. Tomin and W.L. Donegan, Screening for recurrent breast cancer–its effectiveness and prognostic value, *J Clin Oncol* **5** (1987), 62–67.

[10] H.B. Muss, G.S. Tell, L.D. Case, P. Robertson and B.M. Atwell, Perceptions of follow-up care in women with breast cancer, *Am J Clin Oncol* **14** (1991), 55–59.

[11] P. Valagussa, J.D. Tess, A. Rossi, G. Tancini, A. Banfi and G. Bonadonna, Adjuvant CMF effect on site of first recurrence, and appropriate follow- up intervals, in operable breast cancer with positive axillary nodes, *Breast Cancer Res Treat* **1** (1981), 349–356.

[12] E.F. Scanlon, M.A. Oviedo, M.P. Cunningham, J.A. Caprini, J.D. Khandekar, E. Cohen et al., Preoperative and follow-up procedures on patients with breast cancer, *Cancer* **46** (1980), 977–979.

[13] R. Qazi, J.L. Chuang and W. Drobyski, Estrogen receptors and the pattern of relapse in breast cancer, *Arch Intern Med* **144** (1984), 2365–2567.

[14] F.C. Campbell, R.W. Blamey, C.W. Elston, R.I. Nicholson, K. Griffiths and J.L. Haybittle, Oestrogen-receptor status and sites of metastasis in breast cancer, *Br J Cancer* **44** (1981), 456–459.

[15] M. Harris, A. Howell, M. Chrissohou, R.I. Swindell, M. Hudson and R.A. Sellwood, A comparison of the metastatic pattern of infiltrating lobular carcinoma and infiltrating duct carcinoma of the breast, *Br J Cancer* **50** (1984), 23–30.

[16] J. Lamovec and A. Zidar, Association of leptomeningeal carcinomatosis in carcinoma of the breast with infiltrating lobular carcinoma. An autopsy study, *Arch Pathol Lab Med* **115** (1991), 507–510.

[17] A. Ahr, U. Holtrich, C. Solbach, A. Scharl, K. Strebhardt, T. Karn et al., Molecular classification of breast cancer patients by gene expression profiling, *J Pathol* **195** (2001), 312–320.

[18] A. Ahr, T. Karn, C. Solbach, T. Seiter, K. Strebhardt, U. Holtrich et al., Identification of high risk breast-cancer patients by gene expression profiling, *Lancet* **359** (2002), 131–132.

[19] L.J. van 't Veer, H. Dai, M.J. van de Vijver, Y.D. He, A.A. Hart, M. Mao et al., Gene expression profiling predicts clinical outcome of breast cancer, *Nature* **415** (2002), 530–536.

[20] M.J. van de Vijver, Y.D. He, L.J. van't Veer, H. Dai, A.A. Hart, D.W. Voskuil et al., A gene-expression signature as a predictor of survival in breast cancer, *N Engl J Med* **347** (2002), 1999–2009.

[21] E. Hannisdal, S. Gundersen, S. Kvaloy, M.W. Lindegaard, M. Aas, A.M. Finnanger et al., Follow-up of breast cancer patients stage I-II: a baseline strategy, *Eur J Cancer* **7** (1993), 992–997.

[22] A.F. Jacobson, E.B. Cronin, P.C. Stomper and W.D. Kaplan, Bone scans with one or two new abnormalities in cancer patients with no known metastases: frequency and serial scintigraphic behavior of benign and malignant lesions, *Radiology* **175** (1990), 229–232.

[23] R.L. Wahl, R.L. Cody, G.D. Hutchins, E.E. Mudgett, Primary and metastatic breast carcinoma: initial clinical evaluation with PET with the radiolabeled glucose analogue 2-[F-18]-fluoro-2-deoxy- D-glucose, *Radiology* **179** (1991), 765–770.

[24] R.L. Wahl, R. Cody, G. Hutchins and E. Mudgett, Positron-emission tomographic scanning of primary and metastatic breast carcinoma with the radiolabeled glucose analogue 2-deoxy-2-[18F]fluoro- D-glucose, *N Engl J Med* **324** (1991), 200.

[25] R.W. Carlson, Biomarkers in the Surveillance of Early Breast Cancer, *Seminars in Breast Disease* (1999), 2.

[26] M. Gion, R. Mione, A.E. Leon and R. Dittadi, Comparison of the diagnostic accuracy of CA27.29 and CA15.3 in primary breast cancer, *Clin Chem* **45** (1999), 630–637.

[27] D.W. Chan, R.A. Beveridge, H. Muss, H.A. Fritsche, G. Hortobagyi, R. Theriault et al., Use of Truquant BR radioimmunoassay for early detection of breast cancer recurrence in patients with stage II and stage III disease, *J Clin Oncol* **15** (1997), 2322–2328.

[28] C.S. Liu, Y.Y. Shen, C.C. Lin, R.F. Yen and C.H. Kao, Clinical impact of [(18)F]FDG-PET in patients with suspected recurrent breast cancer based on asymptomatically elevated tumor

marker serum levels: a preliminary report, *Jpn J Clin Oncol* **32** (2002), 244–247.

[29] W. Jager, The early detection of disseminated (metastasized) breast cancer by serial tumour marker measurements, *Eur J Cancer Prev* **2**(Suppl 3) (1993), 133–139.

[30] R.C. Bast, Jr., P. Ravdin, D.F. Hayes, S. Bates, H. Fritsche, Jr., J.M. Jessup et al., 2000 update of recommendations for the use of tumor markers in breast and colorectal cancer: clinical practice guidelines of the American Society of Clinical Oncology, *J Clin Oncol* **19** (2001), 1865–1878.

[31] E. Grunfeld, D. Mant, P. Yudkin, R. Adewuyi-Dalton, D. Cole, J. Stewart et al., Routine follow up of breast cancer in primary care: randomised trial, *BMJ* **313** (1996), 665–669.

[32] J. Maher, J. Bradburn and R. Adewuyi-Dalton, Follow up in breast cancer. Patients prefer specialist follow up, *Bmj* **311** (1995), 54.

[33] M.S. Simon, M. Stano, M. Hussein, M. Hoff and D. Smith, An analysis of the cost of clinical surveillance after primary therapy for women with early stage invasive breast cancer, *Breast Cancer Res Treat* **37** (1996), 39–47.

[34] T.J. Smith, N.E. Davidson, D.V. Schapira, E. Grunfeld, H.B. Muss, V.G. Vogel 3rd, et al., American Society of Clinical Oncology 1998 update of recommended breast cancer surveillance guidelines, *J Clin Oncol* **17** (1999), 1080–1082.

[35] R.W. Carlson, B.O. Anderson, W. Bensinger, C.E. Cox, N.E. Davidson, S.B. Edge et al., NCCN Practice Guidelines for Breast Cancer, *Oncology (Huntingt)* **14** (2000), 33–49.

[36] M. Hugi, I. Olivotto, A. Lees et al., Follow-up after treatment of breast cancer, *Can Med Assoc J* **158**(Suppl 3S70) (1998).

[37] N.B.C.C. Australia, National Breast Cancer Center, Clinical Practice Guidelines for the Management of Early Breast Cancer Follow-up. http://nbcc.org/au/pages/info/resource/nbccpubs/clinprof/followup.htm. Accessed Dec. 2002.

[38] ESMO Minimum Clinical Recommendations for diagnosis, adjuvant treatment and follow-up of primary breast cancer, *Ann Oncol* **12** (2001), 1047–1048.

Breast Disease 21 (2004) 55–64
IOS Press

Long-Term Complications of Adjuvant Chemotherapy for Early Stage Breast Cancer

Ann H. Partridge and Eric P. Winer*
Dana-Farber Cancer Institute, Brigham and Women's Hospital, Harvard Medical School, Boston, MA, USA

Abstract. The benefits of adjuvant chemotherapy for early stage breast cancer must be considered in light of the potential risks and anticipated side effects. When considering a course of adjuvant chemotherapy for a patient, one should not only consider acute side effects of treatment, but should understand the long-term risks of therapy. Sustained or long-term effects of adjuvant chemotherapy usually have either a late onset or a sustained impact – often lasting for many years. In the case of some of the rare long-term complications, many years may elapse before any symptoms develop. This review details sustained and long-term complications of adjuvant chemotherapy including information about risk factors, etiology, and incidence rates for specific complications. Interventions to ameliorate long-term complications are also addressed.

INTRODUCTION

Adjuvant chemotherapy significantly improves disease free and overall survival in women with early stage breast cancer [1]. However, the benefits of adjuvant therapy must be considered in light of the potential risks and anticipated side effects. Side effects from treatment can be divided according to when they most commonly occur. Acute side effects typically occur during the course of treatment and generally resolve within months of the completion of therapy. By contrast, sustained or long-term effects usually have either a later onset or a more sustained impact – often lasting for many years. In the case of some of the rare long-term complications, many years may elapse before any symptoms develop.

Adjuvant breast cancer chemotherapy may give rise to a number of sustained or long-term complications. Table 1 lists the possible long-term effects of adjuvant chemotherapy. Some of these complications are extremely rare, such as secondary leukemia. Others, such as premature ovarian failure or weight gain, are seen

much more commonly. Some complications are regimen specific, as is the case of cardiac dysfunction following treatment with anthracycline-based chemotherapy. Other effects may depend less on the specific regimen but are seen more commonly in specific patient subgroups, such as premature menopause in women over age forty. It is often difficult to predict which individual patients will experience specific complications.

Premature Menopause and Sequellae

Chemotherapy-related amenorrhea or premature menopause is a common consequence of adjuvant chemotherapy in premenopausal women. Amenorrhea occurs because of chemotherapy-induced destruction of maturing ovarian follicles [2]. This results in significant decreases in circulating estrogen and progesterone levels, with subsequent elevation in gonadotrophic hormones, FSH and LH. Because women have a finite number of primordial ovarian follicles, if these are reduced below the minimum number necessary for menstrual cycling, permanent ovarian failure occurs resulting in menopause. Although these changes are similar to the hormonal changes of natural menopause, they may occur more precipitously in women with chemotherapy-related amenorrhea or menopause, resulting in menopausal symptoms that may develop

---

*Corresponding author: Eric P. Winer MD, Breast Oncology Center, Dana-Farber Cancer Institute, 44 Binney Street, Boston, MA 02115, USA. Tel.: +1 617 632 3800; Fax: +1 617 632 2616; E-mail ewiner@partners.org.

more rapidly and be more severe than those associated with natural menopause.

Although most complications of adjuvant therapy are difficult to predict for a given individual, chemotherapy-related amenorrhea is the most predictable as it appears to be a function of patient age, the specific chemotherapeutic agents used, and the total dose administered. The impact of treatment duration and dose intensity, independent of total dose, is uncertain. Table 2 shows the proportion of women who experience premature menopause with adjuvant chemotherapy [3]. The table is divided by treatment regimen and age. In women under the age of 30, premature ovarian failure with any of the available regimens is distinctly uncommon. Three separate reports have provided estimates of 20% or less [4–6]. In two of these studies [4,6], there were no patients under age 30 who experienced premature menopause. Goodwin and colleagues evaluated the incidence of ovarian failure in women who received no systemic therapy compared to those who received either chemotherapy or chemotherapy followed by tamoxifen [7]. Young women (under the age of 30) had a very low incidence of menopause regardless of the therapy received. As expected, the incidence of chemotherapy-related amenorrhea increased with age. The vast majority of women over the age of 40 experience ovarian failure after treatment with CMF or CEF. In women under the age of 40, the risk of ovarian failure from these regimens is lower and declines with decreasing age. MF has been reported to be associated with an approximately 10% incidence of premature menopause, but this has not been analyzed as a function of patient age. AC is associated with a lower incidence of premature menopause in both younger and older women, probably because of the lower cumulative dose of cyclophosphamide and anthracycline with this regimen. The effect of adjuvant taxane therapy on the ovaries has not yet been well evaluated. In one small retrospective study, the addition of paclitaxel to AC did not appear to substantially increase the overall risk of chemotherapy related amenorrhea [8], however larger studies are needed to make any definitive conclusions.

It is important to note that some women will resume menstrual function months or years after treatment. However, the vast majority of women who remain amenorrheic one year following treatment will not regain ovarian function. The possibility of late but nevertheless premature menopause has not been thoroughly explored. There is evidence that adolescent girls who received chemotherapy for pediatric cancers may experience an earlier that expected

menopause [9]. It is not clear whether a premenopausal woman who receives chemotherapy and does not experience chemotherapy-related amenorrhea at that time will go through menopause earlier than she would have in the absence of chemotherapy.

While premature menopause may have a beneficial effect on breast cancer prognosis in women with hormone receptor-positive tumors [10], early menopause may cause significant physiologic and psychosocial consequences. For women who are interested in becoming pregnant after breast cancer, the risk of infertility following adjuvant chemotherapy is an important concern and may impact on decision making. For many women, menopausal symptoms such as hot flashes, genitourinary problems, and both psychological and sexual difficulties are a significant problem following adjuvant chemotherapy [11–13]. Some of these symptoms or complications may be ameliorated with hormonal or non-hormonal interventions [14–16].

Premature ovarian failure may also contribute to increased cardiovascular morbidity, though data to support this concern in women with breast cancer are lacking. In addition, women who experience premature menopause also have accelerated loss of bone mineral density and may develop osteoporosis [17–21]. Shapiro et al. [21] evaluated bone mineral density at baseline and in follow-up of forty-nine premenopausal women with early stage breast cancers receiving adjuvant chemotherapy. Among the 35 women who were defined as having experienced ovarian failure during therapy, they observed highly significant bone loss in the lumbar spine by 6 months and increased further at 12 months. The median percentage decrease of bone mineral density in the spine from 0 to 6 months and 6 to 12 months was -4.0 (range, -10.4 to $+1.0$; $P = 0.0001$) and -3.7 (range, -10.1 to 9.2; $P = 0.0001$), respectively. In contrast, there were no significant decreases in bone mineral density in the 14 patients who retained ovarian function. In addition, markers of skeletal turnover including serum osteocalcin and bone specific alkaline phosphatase increased significantly in the women who developed ovarian failure. Based on these findings women with breast cancer who develop chemotherapy-induced ovarian failure may be at higher risk for osteopenia, and subsequently osteoporosis, and should consider having their bone density monitored. Among women with hormone receptor-positive tumors, bone loss may be offset to some degree by the use of tamoxifen, through its proestrogenic effects [22,23]. In addition, there are several available non-hormonal interventions to attenuate bone loss [14–16].

Table 1
Sustained and Long-term complications of adjuvant chemotherapy for breast cancer

Common Complications (> 10% of patients develop)
– Premature Menopause*/Infertility
– Osteoporosis
– Weight Gain*
– QOL Issues*
Extremely Rare Complications (< 2% of patients develop)
– Cardiac Dysfunction
– Leukemia/Myelodysplastic Syndrome
Additional Complications
– Neuropathy*- incidence of long-term effects uncertain
– Cognitive Dysfunction- preliminary evidence from cross-sectional studies only

*May be both acute and long-term effects.

Table 2
Risk of premature menopause by regimen and age

		Incidence of amenorrhea (%)	
Regimen	Duration (mos.)	age < 40 yr	age ⩾ 40 yr
CMF-based	6	30–40%	80–96%
	12	50–80%	80–98%
FEC*	6	20–25%	>85%
AC*	3	<15%	50–70%
MF	6	~10%	

Adapted with permission from Burstein and Winer in J.R. Harris' Diseases of the Breast, 2000 [3].
*In some series, no women under 30 developed chemotherapy-induced premature menopause following standard anthracycline-based chemotherapy [4,6,7].

Weight Gain

Weight gain is a common complaint among women who have received adjuvant chemotherapy. It has been reported in 50% or more of women following adjuvant chemotherapy, with mean gains of 2.5–5.0 kg [24–27]. In as many as 20% of patients, more significant weight gain, as much as 10–20 kg, has been reported. Risk of weight gain appears to be related to menopausal status, incidence of premature menopause, and duration of chemotherapy. Weight gain is more common among premenopausal than postmenopausal women, with women who experience menopause with chemotherapy at greater risk [24–26]. Regimens that are longer in duration also may increase the risk of weight gain, and weight gain may be less common with the shorter AC regimen [28].

The underlying cause of weight gain with chemotherapy is uncertain and had been assumed to occur because women receiving chemotherapy simply increased their food consumption. However, studies monitoring dietary intake have failed to support this hypothesis [26,29,30]. Recent data suggests that weight gain may be due to decreased physical activity during ther-

apy [28–30]. There have been conflicting data with regard whether or not chemotherapy has an effect on resting metabolic rate. Some studies have suggested that resting metabolic rate may decrease, and that lean body mass can decline following a course of chemotherapy [27–31], although other investigators have failed to confirm this finding [32].

Weight gain can have an enormous influence on a woman's physical health and psychosocial adaptation following adjuvant chemotherapy. In addition, retrospective studies have suggested that weight gain may increase a woman's risk of disease recurrence [33–36]. Interventions focusing on exercise and increasing lean body mass may help to ameliorate weight gain among women receiving adjuvant breast cancer chemotherapy [30].

Quality of Life Issues

Adjuvant chemotherapy may have a profound impact on a woman's overall quality of life (QOL). For the majority of women, QOL appears to worsen during adjuvant therapy followed by definite improvement after completion of therapy [37]. Some women, however, may continue to experience poor QOL for an extended period following adjuvant chemotherapy. Broeckel et al., surveyed 61 disease-free breast cancer survivors who had completed adjuvant chemotherapy an average of 16 months earlier (range 3–36 months) and compared them to 59 age-matched controls with no history of cancer [38]. The breast cancer survivors scored more poorly than the noncancer comparison group on a measure of depression (CES-D) and on six of the eight subscales of a quality of life measure (SF-36). Younger age, being unmarried, shorter interval since cancer diagnosis and chemotherapy all predicted greater depressive symptomatology ($p < 0.05$). Physical well-being was not predicted by any of the demographic or medical variables assessed. Ganz and colleagues evaluated 763 breast cancer survivors who remained disease-free an average of 6.3 years from diagnosis regarding their QOL [39]. Overall, they found that physical and emotional well-being was excellent with survivors reporting high levels of functioning and QOL. Of note, in a multivariate analysis, women who had not received systemic adjuvant therapy had a better current QOL than those who had previously received systemic adjuvant therapy (chemotherapy, tamoxifen, or both together) ($P = 0.003$). These data suggest that there may be a persistent impact of adjuvant treatment on QOL.

Fatigue has been recognized increasingly in recent years as a common side effect of cancer chemotherapy. Fatigue has been shown to have a negative impact on overall QOL in breast cancer survivors [40,41]. For most women, fatigue improves following the cessation of therapy, however, there is growing evidence that a substantial minority of patients may have difficulty with fatigue for months and even years following adjuvant chemotherapy [40,42–45].

Women may also experience long-term sexual dysfunction following breast cancer treatment which may have a negative impact on a woman's QOL. Women who have received adjuvant chemotherapy may be particularly at risk [46–48]. Sexual difficulties may be amenable to interventions to improve functioning. In one study, 76 postmenopausal breast cancer survivors with at least one severe menopausal symptom (i.e., hot flashes, vaginal dryness, and stress urinary incontinence) were randomized to either to usual-care or an intervention focused on symptom assessment, education, counseling and, as appropriate, specific pharmacologic and behavioral interventions for specific symptoms [49]. After a 4 month period during which the intervention took place, patients receiving the intervention demonstrated statistically significant improvement

in menopausal symptoms ($P = 0.0004$) and sexual functioning ($P = 0.04$) compared with the usual-care group.

Cognitive Dysfunction

Cognitive dysfunction after adjuvant therapy has received increasing attention in both the medical and lay literature in recent years. Anecdotally, many women report difficulties with concentration and memory while receiving and after completing adjuvant chemotherapy. There are multiple factors that may contribute to difficulties with cognitive function during this time including psychosocial distress, antiemetic medications, hormonal changes, and fatigue. Three cross-sectional studies have compared cognitive function in women who received chemotherapy and a control group [50–52]. All of these studied used detailed neuropsychiatric testing to evaluate study participants. Schagen et al. evaluated 39 women who were approximately two years out from 6 cycles of CMF (with or without subsequent tamoxifen) and compared them to 34 women who had received local therapy only [51]. Twenty-eight percent of the CMF group compared to 12% of the controls had evidence of cognitive dysfunction, predominantly characterized by difficulties with concentration, memory, word-finding, and motor testing. Hormonal therapy did not appear to influence patients' self-reports of symptoms or cognitive function. In a study by van Dam and colleagues, a dose-effect relationship was seen between chemotherapy and cognitive dysfunction [50,53]. At a mean of 2 years since the completion of last nonhormonal therapy, impaired cognitive dysfunction was seen in 32% of the patients treated with high dose chemotherapy, in 17% of the patients treated with standard dose chemotherapy, and in 9% of women with stage I breast cancer who did not receive chemotherapy. Brezden et al. surveyed a group of 31 women receiving chemotherapy, another group of 40 women who had received chemotherapy in the past, and a group of healthy controls [52]. Impaired cognition was seen more frequently in women on active treatment compared to controls, and cognitive difficulties did not appear to be related to anxiety or depression. While these results are provocative, it is important to note that in two of the studies, there was no association between self-reports of cognitive dysfunction and scores on the formal testing; the women who complained of cognitive difficulties were not the same women who performed poorly on the testing [50, 51].

More recently, studies evaluating long-term cognitive functioning after adjuvant therapy have yielded conflicting results. Ahles and colleagues evaluated long-term cognitive functioning in survivors of breast cancer and lymphoma [54]. Among 71 patients who were, on average, over 10 years out from treatment, survivors who had been treated with systemic chemotherapy scored significantly lower on the battery of neuropsychologic tests than those treated with local therapy only ($P < 0.04$), particularly in the domains of verbal memory ($P < 0.01$) and psychomotor functioning ($P < 0.03$). Survivors treated with systemic chemotherapy were also more likely to score in the lower quartile on the Neuropsychological Performance Index (39% v 14%, $P < 0.01$) and to self-report greater problems with working memory ($P < 0.02$). Schagen et al. performed a follow-up longitudinal study of breast cancer survivors comparing those who had received local therapy only to women who had receive either high dose therapy, FEC, or CMF. In this study, at 4 years follow-up, improvement in performance was observed in all chemotherapy groups, whereas in the control group there was a slight deterioration in test results. These findings would suggest that cognitive dysfunction following adjuvant chemotherapy in breast cancer patients may be transient.

The possibility of persistent impaired cognition is of great concern to women who are making decisions about adjuvant treatment. At the present time, firm conclusions cannot be made about the incidence, impact or duration of cognitive dysfunction following adjuvant chemotherapy. Prospective longitudinal studies are ongoing to further evaluate and characterize changes in cognitive function in women following adjuvant chemotherapy, as well as to evaluate potential preventative measures [55,56].

Neuropathy

With the incorporation of the taxanes into adjuvant chemotherapy regimens, peripheral neuropathy- both sensory and motor- has been seen increasingly. Severity of neuropathy appears to be related to individual dose, cumulative dose, and schedule of administration [57]. Although neuropathy is usually mild to moderate and resolves spontaneously following discontinuation of the drug, it can be a chronic complaint for some patients following taxane chemotherapy [58,59]. In Cancer and Leukemia Group B (CALGB) Protocol 9344 in which patients were randomized to AC or AC followed by 4 cycles of paclitaxel, only 3% of patients

who received paclitaxel developed sensory neurotoxicity that interfered with normal functioning, while 15% of patients had moderate parasthesias [60]. The preliminary report of the Breast Cancer International Research Group (BCIRG) study of docetaxel, adriamycin and cyclophosphamide (TAC) vs. 5-fluorouracil, adriamycin and cyclophosphamide (FAC) did not report grade 3 or 4 neuropathy as a side effect that occurred in 5% of women or more [61].

In the preliminary report of the Intergroup C9741 Protocol, in which women on all three arms received four cycles of paclitaxel at 175 mg/m^2 each, the incidence of severe sensory loss or motor weakness was < 5% in all arms [62]. The incidence of long-term neurologic sequellae after adjuvant chemotherapy is currently unknown and several ongoing trials incorporating the taxanes should further elucidate the risk. A variety of interventions are under evaluation to prevent or ameliorate neuropathic effects of chemotherapy.

Late Cardiac Effects

Cardiotoxicity is one of the most worrisome risks of adjuvant chemotherapy and has been a major concern as anthracycline-based regimens have been used more commonly in the adjuvant setting. Fortunately, the incidence of clinically significant cardiac impairment is rare, developing in less than 2% of women receiving standard adjuvant anthracycline-based regimens. The incidence of anthracycline-induced cardiac dysfunction increases with increasing cumulative amount of anthracycline (either doxorubicin or epirubicin) administered. Other risk factors include advancing age, and underlying cardiac disease [63,64]. In general, most adjuvant chemotherapy regimens restrict cumulative doses of doxorubicin to less than 360 mg/m^2 and epirubicin to less than 720 mg/m^2, doses thought to fall within a relatively safe range with clinically acceptable rates of cardiac complication. Valagussa et al. reported a 0.8% incidence of congestive heart failure (CHF) in a group of over 500 women who received approximately 250 mg/m^2 of doxorubicin, with a median follow-up of 80 months [65]. Zambetti and colleagues performed a more detailed long-term assessment of cardiac function in a group of 355 women who were disease free at a median follow-up of 11.5 years [66]. Fifty-six percent of women received CMF followed by doxorubicin, with a median cumulative doxorubicin dose of approximately 300 mg/m^2, and 44% percent received CMF only. Although clinical CHF was very rare in both groups, 8% of the women in the doxorubicin group were characterized as having systolic dysfunction, defined as an ejection fraction of less than 55%, in comparison to less than 2% of the CMF group developing evidence of systolic dysfunction. In a recent US Intergroup trial using 6 cycles of CAF chemotherapy in postmenopausal women, the reported incidence of CHF was approximately 2% [67]. Of note, the patient population was somewhat older than in many adjuvant trials and the total planned dose of doxorubicin was 360 mg/m^2.

For women receiving anthracycline-based therapy in the adjuvant setting, prophylactic measures are not routinely taken to prevent cardiac damage as the risk is very small. Nevertheless, selected centers have chosen to administer adriamycin as a prolonged continuous infusion to minimize the risk of cardiotoxicity. In women with baseline cardiac dysfunction or those who are at risk for compromise based on their medical history, it is prudent to evaluate cardiac function prior to initiating anthracycline-based adjuvant therapy. Although the available data are reassuring, it remains unknown whether previous anthracycline exposure increases the risk of cardiac compromise with a subsequent cardiac event (e.g. a myocardial infarction).

There has also been speculation that left-sided breast/chest wall irradiation increases the risk of cardiac toxicity in the setting of anthracycline-based adjuvant chemotherapy. In a randomized trial of 5 vs. 10 cycles of CA, the increased risk of cardiac events in the women who received 10 courses of treatment (median cumulative dose of doxorubicin 442 mg/m^2) was more pronounced in women who also received high dose-volume of cardiac irradiation [68]. There appeared to be no excess cardiac risk in women who received 5 cycles of AC (median cumulative dose of doxorubicin 225 mg/m^2) with radiation. In a retrospective analysis from Valagussa et al., a total of 4 of 501 women (0.8%) treated with doxorubicin had developed congestive heart failure by a median follow-up in excess of 6 years [65]. Of the 114 women who received doxorubicin and left-sided breast irradiation, 3 women developed heart failure (2.6%). With the availability of modern radiation planning, minimizing cardiac volume in the radiation field, the risk of left-sided irradiation and the use of doxorubicin appears to be minimized.

The risk of cardiac dysfunction with the addition of trastuzumab to adjuvant therapy regimens studies is currently under evaluation. In the treatment of metastatic breast cancer, cardiotoxicity has been reported to occur with trastuzumab when administered alone and in combination with antineoplastic agents, particularly anthracyclines [69,70]. The risk of significant cardiotoxicity with trastuzumab monotherapy has been reported to be 3 to 7%, and up to 27% when trastuzumab is administered in combination with an anthracycline and cyclophosphamide [70]. The majority of reported cardiac effects occurring on trastuzumab therapy are mild to moderate, nonspecific, and medically manageable, although they can be life threatening. Unlike classical anthracycline-induced toxicity, trastuzumab-associated toxicity usually responds to standard treatment or the discontinuation of trastuzumab, and there is no evidence that the toxicity is dose related [69–71]. The pathogenesis and histologic changes responsible for trastuzumab-associated cardiotoxicity currently are under investigation [71]. In ECOG protocol 2198, 234 women with stage II breast cancer were randomized to receive 4 cycles of adjuvant paclitaxel plus trastuzumab (TH) prior to 4 cycles of doxorubicin and cyclophosphamide (AC) or to the same regimen followed by 52 weeks trastuzumab and cardiac function was evaluated serially in both groups [72]. In this study, decreases in left-ventricular ejection fraction (LVEF) > 10% from baseline levels were seen in 18 of 189 of patients (9.5%) post-TH, and in 16 of 128 patients (12.5%) post-AC. Drops in LVEF below the lower limit of normal were seen in 4 of 189 patients post-TH, and in 7 of 128 patients post-AC. Grade 3/4 cardiac toxicity was seen in 8 patients (7 grade 3, 1 grade 4) in the entire study, with one case of CHF reported post-TH. In a single institution study of 40 patients with stage 2 or 3 breast cancer receiving preoperative trastuzumab and herceptin, with subsequent adjuvant doxorubicin and cyclophosphamide chemotherapy following definitive breast surgery, LVEF was measured at baseline, after 12 weeks of neoadjuvant paclitaxel and trastuzumab, and following cycles 2 and 4 of AC chemotherapy [73]. During the neoadjuvant phase of therapy, four patients had grade 1 decline in LVEF, and one patient had a grade 2 decrease. All these patients continued on with adjuvant therapy. During the adjuvant AC phase of therapy, five patients were observed to have grade 1 toxicity, and four patients had grade 2 toxicity. No patients developed symptomatic (grade 3 or 4) heart failure. While the absence of clinical cardiac toxicity is reassuring, ongoing adjuvant studies incorporating trastuzumab are monitoring closely for potential cardiotoxicity, evaluating cardiac function at baseline and regularly during treatment by physical examination and measurement of LVEF.

Chemotherapy-Associated Leukemia

Leukemia or myelodysplastic syndrome (MDS) following adjuvant chemotherapy is an extremely rare, usually life-threatening complication of treatment. In early studies, the total dose of cyclophosphamide emerged as an important risk factor, with a substantially higher risk in women who receive more than 20,000 mg of the drug. Curtis et al. conducted a case-control study of 82,700 women treated for breast cancer during the 1970's and 80's [74]. Based on this study, the investigators estimated that typical CMF regimens, which utilize relatively low cumulative doses of cyclophosphamide, were estimated to cause an additional 5 cases of leukemia than would be seen baseline in 10,000 women over 10 years. The incidence of leukemia or MDS in women after standard dose adjuvant therapy with anthracycline-based regimens, may be greater than with classical CMF, with reported rates ranging from approximately 0.1–1.5% at 5–10 years follow-up [67, 75–83].

In clinical trials using 6 months of an adjuvant anthracycline and cyclophosphamide containing regimen (CEF, FAC), the incidence of leukemia or MDS has been found to be as high as 1.5% [75,77], with an even greater risk for women who also received radiation therapy [75]. Following 4 cycles of standard CA chemotherapy (cyclophosphamide 600 mg/m^2 and doxorubicin 60 mg/m^2 per cycle), the risk appears quite low. In one study, the incidence of leukemia or MDS in women who receive 4 cycles of CA was 0.1% with a median follow-up of 5 years [76]. By contrast, women had a higher risk of leukemia and MDS in NSABP protocols B-22 and B-25 using higher dose cyclophosphamide in combination with doxorubicin and supported by G-CSF [76,82]. In both studies, there was no benefit in disease-free or overall survival observed among women who received the higher dose therapy, and rates of leukemia and MDS ranged from 0.1–1.2%. It is hypothesized that the higher doses of cyclophosphamide, up to 2400 mg/m^2 per cycle, may have contributed to the higher incidence of leukemia and MDS in these studies. To date, there does not appear to be additional risk of leukemia or MDS with the incorporation of the taxanes into the adjuvant setting. In CALGB 9344, in which women were randomized to receive either 4 cycles of AC followed by paclitaxel (T) vs. AC alone (with A dose escalation), there were no significant differences in the incidence of leukemia and MDS on any of the study arms with an overall reported incidence of 0.5% [60]. In the preliminary report of the NSABP B-28 trial, 5 cases of leukemia developed in the approximately 1500 patients who received standard dose AC followed by paclitaxel (approximately 0.3% incidence) [84]. At 4 years median follow-up, there

has been no differential risk of leukemia or MDS seen in the recently reported Intergroup C9741 trial of AC followed by paclitaxel administered every 2 weeks with G-CSF support compared with every 3 week administration [62].

The latency period and cytogenetic abnormalities appear to be different with anthracycline-induced leukemia or MDS than those that arise after exposure to cyclophosphamide alone [81]. Leukemia or MDS following exposure to topoisomerase inhibitors, such as anthracyclines, tend to occurs from six months to five years after therapy. Leukemia following exposure to alkylating agents, such as cyclophosphamide, typically present five to seven years after treatment and are frequently preceded by a myelodysplastic syndrome.

There are no methods of screening for secondary leukemia or MDS in survivors of breast cancer. However, evaluation should be considered in patients with unexplained cytopenias following adjuvant therapy. Concern about this very rare complication of adjuvant breast cancer chemotherapy seems most reasonable in women who are at low risk of breast cancer recurrence and are likely to derive a very small benefit from adjuvant chemotherapy.

Conclusions

In summary, there are an array of sustained or long-term complications that may result from adjuvant breast cancer chemotherapy and should be considered when assisting women who are making treatment decisions. Some outcomes, such as premature menopause, are predictable for a given individual and many are not. For many complications, there are pharmacotherapeutic and/or psychosocial interventions available or under evaluation which may ameliorate symptoms or prevent future complications. The impact of adjuvant therapy on aspects of quality of life has been increasingly studied. Somewhat surprisingly, it appears that adjuvant treatment may have adverse effects on quality of life in some women even many years following therapy. Serious medical complications resulting from adjuvant chemotherapy including leukemia and congestive heart failure are extremely rare and should be considered very carefully when evaluating the risks and benefits of adjuvant chemotherapy for an individual woman with breast cancer.

REFERENCES

[1] Polychemotherapy for early breast cancer: an overview of the randomised trials. Early Breast Cancer Trialists' Collaborative Group, *Lancet* **352** (1998), 930–942.

[2] M.L. Meistrich, R. Vassilopoulou-Sellin and L.I. Lipshultz, Gonadal Dysfunction, in: *Cancer Priciples and Practice of Oncology*, V.T. DeVita, S. Hellman and S.A. Rosenberg, eds, 6th ed. Philadelphia: Lippincott Williams and Wilkins, 2001, pp. 2923–2939.

[3] H.J. Burstein and E.P. Winer, Reproductive Issues, in: *Diseases of the Breast*, 2nd ed., J.R. Harris, ed., Philadelphia: Lippincott Williams & Wilkins, 2000, pp. 1051–1059.

[4] G.N. Hortobagyi, A.U. Buzdar, C.E. Marcus and T.L. Smith, Immediate and long-term toxicity of adjuvant chemotherapy regimens containing doxorubicin in trials at M.D. Anderson Hospital and Tumor Institute, *NCI Monogr* **1** (1986), 105–109.

[5] P. Valagussa, D. De Candis, G. Antonelli and G. Bonadonna, VIII. Women's health perception and breast cancer: issues of fertility, hormone substitution, and cancer prevention, *Recent Results Cancer Res* **140** (1996), 277–283.

[6] B. Weber and E. Luporsi, Ovarian toxicity of breast cancer chemotherapy, *Eur J Cancer* **34**(5) (1998), S42abstract 170.

[7] P.J. Goodwin, M. Ennis, K.I. Pritchard, M. Trudeau and N. Hood, Risk of menopause during the first year after breast cancer diagnosis, *J Clin Oncol* **17** (1999), 2365–2370.

[8] E.R. Stone, R.S. Slack, A. Novielli, M. Ellis, S. Baidas, E. Gelmann et al., Rate of chemotherapy related amenorrhea (CRA) associated with adjuvant adriamycin and cytoxan (AC) and adriamycin and cytoxan followed by taxol (AC+T) in early stage breast cancer, *Breast Cancer Res Treat* (2000), 64,61, abstract 224.

[9] J. Byrne, T.R. Fears, M.H. Gail, D. Pee, R.R. Connelly, D.F. Austin et al., Early menopause in long-term survivors of cancer during adolescence, *Am J Obstet Gynecol* **166** (1992), 788–793.

[10] O. Pagani, A. O'Neill, M. Castiglione, R.D. Gelber, A. Goldhirsch, C.M. Rudenstam et al., Prognostic impact of amenorrhoea after adjuvant chemotherapy in premenopausal breast cancer patients with axillary node involvement: results of the International Breast Cancer Study Group (IBCSG) Trial VI, *Eur J Cancer* **34** (1998), 632–640.

[11] P.A. Ganz, A. Coscarelli, C. Fred, B. Kahn, M.L. Polinsky and L. Petersen, Breast cancer survivors: psychosocial concerns and quality of life, *Breast Cancer Res Treat* **38** (1996), 183–199.

[12] P.A. Ganz, J.H. Rowland, K. Desmond, B.E. Meyerowitz and G.E. Wyatt, Life after breast cancer: understanding women's health-related quality of life and sexual functioning, *J Clin Oncol* **16** (1998), 501–514.

[13] B.E. Meyerowitz, K.A. Desmond, J.H. Rowland, G.E. Wyatt and P.A. Ganz, Sexuality following breast cancer, *J Sex Marital Ther* **25** (1999), 237–250.

[14] H.J. Burstein and E.P. Winer, Primary care for survivors of breast cancer, *N Engl J Med* **343** (2000), 1086–1094.

[15] P.A. Ganz, Menopause and breast cancer: symptoms, late effects, and their management, *Semin Oncol* **28** (2001), 274–283.

[16] D.L. Barton, C. Loprinzi and B. Gostout, Current management of menopausal symptoms in cancer patients, *Oncology* (*Huntingt*) **16** (2002), 67–72, 4; discussion 5–6, 9–80.

[17] E.D. Kreuser, D. Felsenberg, C. Behles, H. Seibt-Jung, M. Mielcarek, V. Diehl et al., Long-term gonadal dysfunction and its impact on bone mineralization in patients following COPP/ABVD chemotherapy for Hodgkin's disease, *Ann Oncol* **3**(4) (1992), 105–110.

[18] P.F. Bruning, M.J. Pit, M. de Jong-Bakker, A. van den Ende, A. Hart and A. van Enk, Bone mineral density after adjuvant chemotherapy for premenopausal breast cancer, *Br J Cancer* **61** (1990), 308–310.

[19] K.H. Park and C.H. Song, Bone mineral density in premenopausal anovulatory women, *J Obstet Gynaecol* **21** (1995), 89–97.

[20] S.J. Howell, G. Berger, J.E. Adams and S.M. Shalet, Bone mineral density in women with cytotoxic-induced ovarian failure, *Clin Endocrinol (Oxf)* **49** (1998), 397–402.

[21] C.L. Shapiro, J. Manola and M. Leboff, Ovarian failure after adjuvant chemotherapy is associated with rapid bone loss in women with early-stage breast cancer, *J Clin Oncol* **19** (2001), 3306–3311.

[22] C.K. Osborne, Tamoxifen in the treatment of breast cancer, *N Engl J Med* **339** (1998), 1609–1618.

[23] B. Fisher, J.P. Costantino, D.L. Wickerham, C.K. Redmond, M. Kavanah, W.M. Cronin et al., Tamoxifen for prevention of breast cancer: report of the National Surgical Adjuvant Breast and Bowel Project P-1 Study, *J Natl Cancer Inst* **90** (1998), 1371–1388.

[24] W. Demark-Wahnefried, E.P. Winer and B.K. Rimer, Why women gain weight with adjuvant chemotherapy for breast cancer, *J Clin Oncol* **11** (1993), 1418–1429.

[25] W. Demark-Wahnefried, B.K. Rimer and E.P. Winer, Weight gain in women diagnosed with breast cancer, *J Am Diet Assoc* **97** (1997), 519–526, 29; quiz 27–28.

[26] P.J. Goodwin, M. Ennis, K.I. Pritchard, D. McCready, J. Koo, S. Sidlofsky et al., Adjuvant treatment and onset of menopause predict weight gain after breast cancer diagnosis, *J Clin Oncol* **17** (1999), 120–129.

[27] A. Aslani, R.C. Smith, B.J. Allen, N. Pavlakis, J.A. Levi, Changes in body composition during breast cancer chemotherapy with the CMF-regimen, *Breast Cancer Res Treat* **57** (1999), 285–290.

[28] C.L. Kutynec, L. McCargar, S.I. Barr and T.G. Hislop, Energy balance in women with breast cancer during adjuvant treatment, *J Am Diet Assoc* **99** (1999), 1222–1227.

[29] W. Demark-Wahnefried, V. Hars, M.R. Conaway, K. Havlin, B.K. Rimer, G. McElveen et al., Reduced rates of metabolism and decreased physical activity in breast cancer patients receiving adjuvant chemotherapy, *Am J Clin Nutr* **65** (1997), 1495–1501.

[30] W. Demark-Wahnefried, B.L. Peterson, E.P. Winer, L. Marks, N. Aziz, P.K. Marcom et al., Changes in weight, body composition, and factors influencing energy balance among premenopausal breast cancer patients receiving adjuvant chemotherapy, *J Clin Oncol* **19** (2001), 2381–2389.

[31] C.L. Cheney, J. Mahloch and P. Freeny, Computerized tomography assessment of women with weight changes associated with adjuvant treatment for breast cancer, *Am J Clin Nutr* **66** (1997), 141–146.

[32] G. Del Rio, S. Zironi, L. Valeriani, R. Menozzi, M. Bondi and M. Bertolini et al., Weight gain in women with breast cancer treated with adjuvant cyclophosphomide, methotrexate and 5-fluorouracil. Analysis of resting energy expenditure and body composition, *Breast Cancer Res Treat* **73** (2002), 267–273.

[33] W.L. Donegan, A.J. Hartz and A.A. Rimm, The association of body weight with recurrent cancer of the breast, *Cancer* **41** (1978), 1590–1594.

[34] R.T. Chlebowski, J.M. Weiner, R. Reynolds, J. Luce, L. Bulcavage and J.R. Bateman, Long-term survival following re-

lapse after 5-FU but not CMF adjuvant breast cancer therapy, *Breast Cancer Res Treat* **7** (1986), 23–30.

[35] J.K. Camoriano, C.L. Loprinzi, J.N. Ingle, T.M. Therneau, J.E. Krook and M.H. Veeder, Weight change in women treated with adjuvant therapy or observed following mastectomy for node-positive breast cancer, *J Clin Oncol* **8** (1990), 1327–1334.

[36] K. Faber-Langendoen, Weight gain in women receiving adjuvant chemotherapy for breast cancer, *Jama* **276** (1996), 855–856.

[37] R.D. Gelber, A. Goldhirsch, C. Hurny, J. Bernhard and R.J. Simes, Quality of life in clinical trials of adjuvant therapies, in: *Consensus Development Conference on the Treatment of Early Stage Breast Cancer*, Washington, DC, Government Printing Office, 1992.

[38] J.A. Broeckel, P.B. Jacobsen, L. Balducci, J. Horton and G.H. Lyman, Quality of life after adjuvant chemotherapy for breast cancer, *Breast Cancer Res Treat* **62** (2000), 141–150.

[39] P.A. Ganz, K.A. Desmond, B. Leedham, J.H. Rowland, B.E. Meyerowitz and T.R. Belin, Quality of life in long-term, disease-free survivors of breast cancer: a follow-up study, *J Natl Cancer Inst* **94** (2002), 39–49.

[40] J.E. Bower, P.A. Ganz, K.A. Desmond, J.H. Rowland, B.E. Meyerowitz and T.R. Belin, Fatigue in breast cancer survivors: occurrence, correlates, and impact on quality of life, *J Clin Oncol* **18** (2000), 743–753.

[41] K.H. Dow, B.R. Ferrell, S. Leigh, J. Ly and P. Gulasekaram, An evaluation of the quality of life among long-term survivors of breast cancer, *Breast Cancer Res Treat* **39** (1996), 261–273.

[42] C. Lindley, S. Vasa, W.T. Sawyer and E.P. Winer, Quality of life and preferences for treatment following systemic adjuvant therapy for early-stage breast cancer, *J Clin Oncol* **16** (1998), 1380–1387.

[43] P.B. Jacobsen and K. Stein, Is Fatigue a Long-term Side Effect of Breast Cancer Treatment? *Cancer Control* **6** (1999), 256–263.

[44] M.A. Andrykowski, S.L. Curran and R. Lightner, Off-treatment fatigue in breast cancer survivors: a controlled comparison, *J Behav Med* **21** (1998), 1–18.

[45] J.A. Broeckel, P.B. Jacobsen, J. Horton, L. Balducci and G.H. Lyman, Characteristics and correlates of fatigue after adjuvant chemotherapy for breast cancer, *J Clin Oncol* **16** (1998), 1689–1696.

[46] P.A. Ganz, J.H. Rowland, K. Desmond, B.E. Meyerowitz and G.E. Wyatt, Life after breast cancer: understanding women's health-related quality of life and sexual functioning, *J Clin Oncol* **16** (1998), 501–514.

[47] C.L. Thors, J.A. Broeckel and P.B. Jacobsen, Sexual functioning in breast cancer survivors, *Cancer Control* **18** (2001), 442–448.

[48] J.A. Broeckel, C.L. Thors, P.B. Jacobsen, M. Small and C.E. Cox, Sexual functioning in long-term breast cancer survivors treated with adjuvant chemotherapy, *Breast Cancer Res Treat* **75** (2002), 241–248.

[49] P.A. Ganz, G.A. Greendale, L. Petersen, L. Zibecchi, B. Kahn and T.R. Belin, Managing menopausal symptoms in breast cancer survivors: results of a randomized controlled trial, *J Natl Cancer Inst* **92** (2000), 1054–1064.

[50] F.S. van Dam, S.B. Schagen, M.J. Muller, W. Boogerd, E. vd Wall, M.E. Droogleever Fortuyn et al., Impairment of cognitive function in women receiving adjuvant treatment for high-risk breast cancer: high-dose versus standard-dose chemotherapy, *J Natl Cancer Inst* **90** (1998), 210–218.

[51] S.B. Schagen, F.S. van Dam, M.J. Muller, W. Boogerd, J. Lindeboom and P.F. Bruning, Cognitive deficits after postoperative adjuvant chemotherapy for breast carcinoma, *Cancer* **85** (1999), 640–650.

[52] C.B. Brezden, K.A. Phillips, M. Abdolell, T. Bunston and I.F. Tannock, Cognitive function in breast cancer patients receiving adjuvant chemotherapy, *J Clin Oncol* **18** (2000), 2695–2701.

[53] P.A. Ganz, Cognitive dysfunction following adjuvant treatment of breast cancer: a new dose-limiting toxic effect? *J Natl Cancer Inst* **90** (1998), 182–183.

[54] T.A. Ahles, A.J. Saykin, C.T. Furstenberg, B. Cole, L.A. Mott, K. Skalla et al., Neuropsychologic impact of standard-dose systemic chemotherapy in long-term survivors of breast cancer and lymphoma, *J Clin Oncol* **20** (2002), 485–493.

[55] J.A. O'Shaughnessy, Effects of epoetin alfa on cognitive function, mood, asthenia, and quality of life in women with breast cancer undergoing adjuvant chemotherapy, *Clin Breast Cancer* **3**(3) (2002), S116–120.

[56] D. Barton and C. Loprinzi, Novel approaches to preventing chemotherapy-induced cognitive dysfunction in breast cancer: the art of the possible, *Clin Breast Cancer* **3**(3) (2002), S121–127.

[57] C.L. Shapiro and A. Recht, Side effects of adjuvant treatment of breast cancer, *N Engl J Med* **344** (2001), 1997–2008.

[58] R.J. Freilich, C. Balmaceda, A.D. Seidman, M. Rubin and L.M. DeAngelis, Motor neuropathy due to docetaxel and paclitaxel, *Neurology* **47** (1996), 115–118.

[59] P.H. Hilkens, J. Verweij, C.J. Vecht, G. Stoter and M.J. van den Bent, Clinical characteristics of severe peripheral neuropathy induced by docetaxel (Taxotere), *Ann Oncol* **8** (1997), 187–190.

[60] I.C. Henderson, D.A. Berry, G.D. Demetri, C.T. Cirrincione, L.J. Goldstein, S. Martino et al., Improved outcomes from adding sequential paclitaxel but not from escalating doxorubicin dose in an adjuvant chemotherapy regimen for patients with node-positive primary breast cancer, *J Clin Oncol* **21** (2003), 1–9.

[61] J. Nabholtz, T. Pienkowski, J. Mackey, M. Pawlicki, J. Guastalla, C. Vogel et al., Phase III trial comparing TAC (docetaxel, doxorubicin, cyclophosphamide) with FAC (5-fluorouracil, doxorubicin, cyclophosphamide) in the adjuvant treatment of node positive breast cancer (BC) patients: interim analysis of the BCIRG 001 study. [Abstract 141], *Proc Am Soc Clin Oncol* (2002), 21:36a.

[62] M. Citron, D. Berry, C. Cirrincione, J. Carpenter, C. Hudis, W. Gradishar et al., Randomized trial of dose-dense versus conventionally scheduled and sequential versus concurrent combination chemotherapy as postoperative adjuvant treatment of node-positive primary breast cancer: First report of Intergroup Trial C9741/Cancer and Leukemia Group B Trial 9741, *J Clin Oncol* **21**(8) (15 April 2003), 1431–1439.

[63] D.D. Von Hoff, M.W. Layard, P. Basa, H.L. Davis, A.L. Von Hoff, M. Rozencweig et al., Risk factors for doxorubicin-induced congestive heart failure, *Ann Intern Med* **91** (1979), 710–717.

[64] P.K. Singal and N. Iliskovic, Doxorubicin-induced cardiomyopathy, *N Engl J Med* **339** (1998), 900–905.

[65] P. Valagussa, M. Zambetti, S. Biasi, A. Moliterni, R. Zucali and G. Bonadonna, Cardiac effects following adjuvant chemotherapy and breast irradiation in operable breast cancer, *Ann Oncol* **5** (1994), 209–216.

[66] M. Zambetti, A. Moliterni, C. Materazzo, M. Stefanelli, S. Cipriani, P. Valagussa et al., Long-Term Cardiac Sequelae in

Operable Breast Cancer Patients Given Adjuvant Chemotherapy With or Without Doxorubicin and Breast Irradiation, *J Clin Oncol* **19** (2001), 37–43.

[67] K. Albain, S. Green, P. Ravdin, E. Cobau, J. Levine, K. Ingle et al., Overall survival after cyclophosphamide, adriamycin, 5-FU, and tamoxifen (CAFT) is superior to T alone in postmenopausal, receptor (+), node (+) breast cancer: new findings from phase III Southwest Oncology Group Intergroup Trial S8814 (INT-0100), *Proc Am Soc Clin Oncol* (2001), 20:24a abstract 94.

[68] C.L. Shapiro, P.H. Hardenbergh, R. Gelman, D. Blanks, P. Hauptman, A. Recht et al., Cardiac effects of adjuvant doxorubicin and radiation therapy in breast cancer patients, *J Clin Oncol* **16** (1998), 3493–3501.

[69] D.J. Slamon, B. Leyland-Jones, S. Shak, H. Fuchs, V. Paton, A. Bajamonde et al., Use of chemotherapy plus a monoclonal antibody against HER2 for metastatic breast cancer that overexpresses HER2, *N Engl J Med* **344** (2001), 783–792.

[70] A. Seidman, C. Hudis, M.K. Pierri, S. Shak, V. Paton, M. Ashby et al., Cardiac dysfunction in the trastuzumab clinical trials experience, *J Clin Oncol* **20** (2002), 1215–1221.

[71] D.L. Keefe, Trastuzumab-associated cardiotoxicity, *Cancer* **95** (2002), 1592–1600.

[72] G.W. Sledge, A. O'Neill, A.D. Thor, S.P. Kahanic, P.J. Zander, N.E. Davidson et al., Pilot trial of paclitaxel-herceptin adjuvant therapy for early stage breast cancer (E2198).[abstract], *Br Cancer Res Treat* (2001), 69:209 abstract 4.

[73] H.J. Burstein, L.N. Harris, R. Gelman, S.C. Lester, R.A. Nunes, C.M. Kaelin et al., Preoperative therapy with trastuzumab and paclitaxel followed by sequential adjuvant doxorubicin/cyclophosphamide for HER2 overexpressing stage II or III breast cancer: a pilot study, *J Clin Oncol* **21** (2003), 46–53.

[74] R.E. Curtis, J.D. Boice, M. Stovall, L. Bernstein, R.S. Greenberg, J.T. Flannery et al., Risk of leukemia after chemotherapy and radiation treatment for breast cancer, *N Engl J Med* **326** (1992), 1745–1751.

[75] E. Diamandidou, A.U. Buzdar, T.L. Smith, D. Frye, M. Witjaksono and G.N. Hortobagyi, Treatment-related leukemia in breast cancer patients treated with fluorouracil-doxorubicin-cyclophosphamide combination adjuvant chemotherapy: the University of Texas M.D. Anderson Cancer Center experience, *J Clin Oncol* **14** (1996), 2722–2730.

[76] B. Fisher, S. Anderson, D.L. Wickerham, A. DeCillis, N. Dimitrov, E. Mamounas et al., Increased intensification and total dose of cyclophosphamide in a doxorubicin-cyclophosphamide regimen for the treatment of primary breast cancer: findings from National Surgical Adjuvant Breast and Bowel Project B-22, *J Clin Oncol* **15** (1997), 1858–1869.

[77] M.N. Levine, V.H. Bramwell, K.I. Pritchard, B.D. Norris, L.E. Shepherd, H. Abu-Zahra et al., Randomized trial of intensive cyclophosphamide, epirubicin, and fluorouracil chemotherapy compared with cyclophosphamide, methotrexate, and fluorouracil in premenopausal women with node-positive breast cancer. National Cancer Institute of Canada Clinical Trials Group [see comments], *J Clin Oncol* **16** (1998), 2651–2658.

[78] G. Chaplain, C. Milan, C. Sgro, P.M. Carli and C. Bonithon-Kopp, Increased risk of acute leukemia after adjuvant chemotherapy for breast cancer: a population-based study, *J Clin Oncol* **18** (2000), 2836–2342.

[79] J. Pedersen-Bjergaard, Acute promyelocytic leukemia with t(15;17) following inhibition of DNA topoisomerase II, *Ann Oncol* **6** (1995), 751–753.

[80] M.S. Tallman, R. Gray, J.M. Bennett, D. Variakojis, N. Robert, W.C. Wood et al., Leukemogenic potential of adjuvant chemotherapy for early-stage breast cancer: the Eastern Cooperative Oncology Group experience, *J Clin Oncol* **13** (1995), 1557–1563.

[81] M.J. Thirman and R.A. Larson, Therapy-related myeloid leukemia, *Hematol Oncol Clin North Am* **10** (1996), 293–320.

[82] B. Fisher, S. Anderson, A. DeCillis, N. Dimitrov, J.N. Atkins, L. Fehrenbacher et al., Further evaluation of intensified and increased total dose of cyclophosphamide for the treatment of primary breast cancer: findings from National Surgical Adjuvant Breast and Bowel Project B-25, *J Clin Oncol* **17** (1999), 3374–3388.

[83] P. Valagussa, A. Moliterni, M. Terenziani, M. Zambetti and G. Bonadonna, Second malignancies following CMF-based adjuvant chemotherapy in resectable breast cancer, *Ann Oncol* **5** (1994), 803–838.

[84] E.P. Mamounas, Evaluating the use of paclitaxel following doxorubicin/cyclophosphamide in patients with breast cancer and postive axillary nodes. Adjuvant Therapy for Breast Cancer- NIH Consensus Development Conferencem, Bethesda, MD: NIH; 2000.